Pediatric Cardiology and Pulmonology

Christine M. Houser

Pediatric Cardiology and Pulmonology

A Practically Painless Review

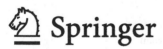 Springer

Christine M. Houser
Department of Emergency Medicine
Erasmus Medical Center
Rotterdam, The Netherlands

ISBN 978-1-4614-9480-5   ISBN 978-1-4614-9481-2 (eBook)
DOI 10.1007/978-1-4614-9481-2
Springer New York Heidelberg Dordrecht London

Library of Congress Control Number: 2013956501

*To my parents Martin and Cathy who made
this journey possible, to Patrick who travels
it with me, and to my wonderful children
Tristan, Skyler, Isabelle, Castiel,
and Sunderland who have patiently
waited during its writing–and are also
the most special of all possible reminders
for why pediatric medicine is so important.*

Important Notice

Medical knowledge and accepted standards of care change frequently. Conflicts are also found regularly in the information provided by various recognized sources in the medical field. Every effort has been made to ensure that the information contained in this publication is as up to date and accurate as possible. However, the parties involved in the publication of this book and its component parts, including the author, the content reviewers, and the publisher, do not guarantee that the information provided is in every case complete, accurate, or representative of the entire body of knowledge for a topic. We recommend that all readers review the current academic medical literature for any decisions regarding patient care.

Preface

Keeping all of the relevant information at your fingertips in a field as broad as pediatrics is both an important task and quite a lot to manage. Add to that the busy schedule most physicians and physicians-to-be carry of practice or studies, family life, and personal obligations, and it can be daunting. Whether you would like to keep your knowledge base up to date for your practice, are preparing for the general pediatric board examination or recertification, or are just doing your best to be well prepared for a ward rotation, *Practically Painless Pediatrics* can be a valuable asset.

Practically Painless Pediatrics brings together the information from several major pediatric board review study guides, and more review conferences than any one physician would ever have time to personally attend, for you to review at your own pace. It's important, especially if there isn't a lot of uninterrupted study time available, to find materials that make the study process as efficient and flexible as possible. What makes this book quite unusual among medical study guides is its design using "bite-sized" chunks of information that can be quickly read and processed. Most information is presented in a question-and-answer (Q & A) format that improves attention and focus and ultimately learning. Critically important for most in medicine, it also enhances the speed with which the information can be learned.

Because the majority of information is in question-and-answer (Q & A) format, it is also much easier to use the information in a few minutes of downtime at the hospital or the office. You don't need to get deeply into the material to understand what you are reading. Each question and answer is brief – not paragraphs long as is often the case in medical review books – which means that the material can be moved through rapidly, keeping the focus on the most critical information.

At the same time, the items have been written to ensure that they contain the necessary information. Very often, the information provided in review books raises as many questions as it answers. This interferes with the study process, because the learner either has to look up the additional information (time loss) or skip the information entirely – therefore not really understanding and learning it. This book keeps answers self-contained, meaning that any needed information is provided either directly in the answer or immediately following it – all without lengthy text.

To provide additional study options, questions and answers are arranged in a simple two-column design, so that it is possible to easily cover one side and quiz yourself or to use the book for quizzing in pairs or study groups.

For a few especially challenging topics, or for the occasional topic that is better presented in a regular text style, a text section has been provided. These sections precede the larger Q & A section for that topic (so, for example, pulmonology text sections will precede the Q & A section for pulmonology). It is important to note that when text sections are present, they are not intended as an overview or an introduction to the Q & A section. They are stand-alone topics found to be more usefully presented as clearly written and relatively brief text sections.

The materials utilized in *Practically Painless Pediatrics* were tested by residents and attendings preparing for the general pediatric board examination, or the recertification examination, to ensure that both the approach and content are on target. All content has also been reviewed by attending and specialist pediatricians to ensure the quality and understandability of the content.

If you are using these materials to prepare for an exam, this can be a great opportunity to thoroughly review some of the many areas involved in pediatric practice and to consolidate and refresh the knowledge developed through the years so far. *Practically Painless Pediatrics* is available to cover the breadth of the topics included in the General Pediatric Board Examination.

This book utilizes the knowledge gained about learning and memory processes over many years of research into cognitive processing. All of us involved in the process of creating it sincerely hope that you will find the study process a bit less onerous with this format and that it becomes at least a times an exciting adventure as you refresh or build your knowledge.

Brief Guidance Regarding the Use of the Book

Items which appear in **bold** indicate topics known to be frequent board examination content. On occasion, an item's content is known to be very specific to previous board questions. In that case, the item will have "popular exam item" beneath it.

At times, you will encounter a Q & A item that covers the same content as a previous item. These items are worded differently and often require you to process the information in a somewhat different way compared to the previous version. This variation in the way questions are asked, for particularly challenging or important content areas, is not an error or an oversight. It is simply a way to easily and automatically practice the information again. These occasional repeat items are designed to increase the probability that the reader will be able to retrieve the information when it is needed – regardless of how the vignette is presented on the exam or how the patient presents in a clinical setting.

Occasionally, a brand name for a medication or a piece of medical equipment is included in the materials. These are indicated with the trademark symbol (®) and are not meant to indicate an endorsement of or recommendation to use that brand name product. Brand names are occasionally included only to make processing of the study items easier, when the brand name is significantly more recognizable to most physicians than the generic name would be.

The specific word choice used in the text may at times seem informal to the reader and occasionally a bit irreverent. Please rest assured that no disrespect is intended to anyone or any discipline, in any case. The mnemonics or the comments provided are only intended to make the material more memorable. The informal wording is often easier to process than the rather complex or unusual wording many of us in the medical field have become accustomed to. That is why rather straightforward wording is sometimes used, even though it may at first seem unsophisticated.

Similarly, visual space is provided on the page, so that the material is not closely crowded together. This improves the ease of using the material for self- or group quizzing and minimizes time potentially wasted identifying which answers belong to which questions.

The reader is encouraged to use the extra space surrounding items to make notes or add comments for himself or herself. Further, the Q & A format is particularly well suited to marking difficult or important items for further review and quizzing. If you are utilizing the book for exam preparation, please consider making a system in advance to indicate which items you'd like to return to, which items have already been repeatedly reviewed, and which items do not require further review. This not only makes the study process more efficient and less frustrating, but it can also offer a handy way to know which items are most important for last-minute review – frequently a very difficult "triage" task as the examination time approaches.

Finally, consider switching back and forth between topics under review to improve processing of new items. Trying to learn and remember many information items on similar topics is often more difficult than breaking the information into chunks by periodically switching to a different topic.

Ultimately, the most important aspect of learning the material needed for board and ward examinations is what we as physicians can bring to our patients – and the amazing gift that patients entrust to us in letting us take an active part in their health. With that focus in mind, the task at hand is not substantially different from what each examination candidate has already done in medical school and in patient care. Keeping that uppermost in our minds, board examination studying should be both a bit less anxiety provoking and a bit more palatable. Seize the opportunity, and happy studying to all!

Rotterdam, The Netherlands   Christine M. Houser

About the Author

Dr. Houser completed her medical degree at the Johns Hopkins University School of Medicine, after spending 4 years in graduate training and research in Cognitive Neuropsychology at George Washington University and the National Institutes of Health (NIH). Her Master of Philosophy degree work focused on the processes involved in learning and memory, and during this time she was a four-time recipient of training awards from the NIH. Dr. Houser's dual interests in cognition and medicine led her naturally toward teaching and "translational cognitive science" – finding ways to apply the many years of cognitive research findings about learning and memory to how physicians and physicians-in-training might more easily learn and recall the vast quantities of information required for medical studies and practice.

Content Reviewers

For Cardiology Topics

Sarosh P. Batlivala, M.D.
Assistant Professor, Pediatric Cardiology
Batson Children's Hospital
University of Mississippi Medical Center
Jackson, MS, USA

Mfon Ekong, M.D.
Assistant Professor of Pediatrics
University of Texas – Houston Medical School
Houston, TX, USA

For Pulmonology Topics

Harish S.R. Rao, M.D.
Assistant Professor
Director of Pediatric Sleep Program
Pennsylvania State Hershey Medical Center
Hershey, PA, USA

Holly D. Smith, M.D.
Assistant Professor of Pediatrics
University of Texas – Houston Medical School
Houston, TX, USA

Latanya J. Love, M.D.
Assistant Professor of Pediatrics and Internal Medicine
University of Texas – Houston Medical School
Houston, TX, USA

Contents

Chapter 1
General Cardiology Question and Answer Items

If the pulse is "bounding," meaning it's noticeably bigger than usual, and falls away faster, too, what are the two most likely causes in children?	1. Large PDA 2. Aortic valve insufficiency
Slow or prolonged rise in the pulse suggests what structural cardiovascular problem?	Aortic stenosis
A midsystolic click at the apex of the heart is probably due to _____?	Mitral valve prolapse
Systolic ejection clicks usually indicate what two types of problems?	1. Thickened or abnormal valves on the aorta or pulmonary artery 2. Bicuspid valves (same vessels)
Which important congenital heart malformations can also cause a systolic ejection click?	1. Truncus arteriosus 2. Tetralogy of Fallot
What is the usual pattern for the S2 heart sound?	• It is split into two sounds • The spacing of the two sounds varies with respiration
If the S2 heart sound is split, but *does not* vary with inspiration, what does that tell you?	It's a "fixed, split, S2"=ASD or pulmonic stenosis (ASD is more common)

C.M. Houser, *Pediatric Cardiology and Pulmonology: A Practically Painless Review*,
DOI 10.1007/978-1-4614-9481-2_1, © Springer Science+Business Media New York 2014

A harsh systolic ejection murmur at the right upper sternal border likely indicates _____?	Aortic valve stenosis
A harsh systolic ejection murmur at the left upper sternal border likely indicates _____?	Pulmonary valve stenosis
VSDs create what sort of murmur?	Holosystolic murmur (usually loud)
The murmur of a patent ductus arteriosus is typically described as _____?	Continuous *Machinery* Murmur
"Egg on a string" heart shape on x-ray is the buzzword for what congenital malformation?	Transposition of the great vessels
A "snowman-" shaped heart is the buzzword for what rare congenital cardiac malformation?	Totally anomalous pulmonary venous return (without obstruction)
Ebstein anomaly, in which the tricuspid valve is malpositioned, is associated with what electrical abnormalities in the heart?	Wolff-Parkinson-White & Right Bundle Branch Block
"Boot-shaped" heart is the famous description of the x-ray appearance of what congenital cardiac malformation?	Tetralogy of Fallot
The hallmark of WPW on EKG is _____?	The delta wave (slurred upstroke to the QRS complex)
If WPW is symptomatic, what is the long-term treatment?	Ablation of the abnormal tissue (usually, but not always, radioablation)
You see a healthy 15-year-old male in the office. He plays a lot of sports and is bradycardic. He has no complaints. On x-ray, his heart is noted to be large. What is the most likely interpretation?	Athletic heart

When should echocardiography be performed for Kawasaki's patient (at minimum)?	1. **At diagnosis** 2. **6–8 weeks later** 3. **6–12 months later**
What CBC finding is a special hallmark of Kawasaki's disease?	**High thrombocytosis (often ≥650)**
What is the risk of coronary aneurysm for Kawasaki's patients who are not treated?	**25 %**
What is the risk of coronary aneurysm for Kawasaki's patients with appropriate management?	**<10 %**
What abdominal/pelvic effects are seen in Kawasaki's Disease?	**Sterile pyuria** **&** **Hydrops of the gallbladder**
Behaviorally, what do you usually see in Kawasaki's patients?	**Significant irritability**
If aortic coarctation is severe, what do you expect to see in the infant?	**Shock and/or CHF**
If a female infant has coarctation of the aorta, what should you check for?	**Turner syndrome**
What x-ray findings are "buzzwords" for aortic coarctation?	**Rib notching** (takes time to develop, seen in older kids & adults) **&** **"3" sign** (the aorta looks like a three due to the constricted part)
What is the simplest way to screen for coarctation?	**Pulses and blood pressure in all extremities**
How is definitive diagnosis of aortic coarctation usually accomplished?	Echocardiography

When a child has mild aortic coarctation, how will it usually present?	Asymptomatic hypertension
Where, and when, will you hear the murmur of aortic coarctation?	Apex and back · Systolic ejection murmur (Remember that murmurs are usually heard where the blood flow is heading, at the spot causing the murmur. Apex & back make sense for a constricted aorta.)
Rheumatic heart disease can occur after what type of infection?	Grp A β-hemolytic strep *pharyngitis* (that wasn't antibiotic treated)
Will rheumatic fever begin during the strep infection?	No – 2–6 weeks later (texts vary – about 4 weeks)
What is the most common cardiac consequence of rheumatic fever?	Mitral valve regurgitation
Which two valves are most often affected by rheumatic fever?	Mitral & aortic (initially regurg, mitral may later develop stenosis)
How is rheumatic fever treated?	Aspirin for pain Steroids if carditis develops Antibiotics for prevention
How is the preventative antibiotic regimen for rheumatic fever given?	IM benzathine PCN G every 28 days (erythromycin for PCN allergic patients)
Using the correct BP cuff is important for obtaining an accurate measure of blood pressure. If the cuff is too small, what will happen to the BP reading?	It will be falsely *high* (too tight, too high)
How do you know if the BP cuff is the correct size?	The air bladder part covers 75% of the upper arm circumference

Hypertension in children is defined as _____?
(Name 2 criteria)

>95% for age
   Or
>2 standard deviations from the mean for age

on *multiple* measurements

Hypertension cannot be diagnosed in a child (or any patient) unless what diagnostic precaution is taken?

Blood pressure is measured multiple times (at least 3!)

(& hypertension criteria are met on the repeated measurements)

The most likely correctable cause of hypertension in a child is _____?

Renal disease

(coarctation is also possible)

What is the significance of an abdominal bruit in a hypertensive child?

Possible renal artery stenosis

What is the first line of treatment for hypertension in pediatrics?

If no correctable cause, then low-salt diet, weight loss, and exercise

What is the second line of treatment for hypertension in pediatrics?

Medication – various types

(β-blockers, Diuretics, ACE inhibitors, Calcium channel blockers)

A patient presents who develops palpitations and chest pain when she/he stands up after being seated for long periods. Family history is positive for unexplained fainting spells. Is this patient nuts? What is the diagnosis?

Not nuts – POTS
Postural Orthostatic Tachycardia Syndrome

Do Postural Orthostasis patients generally have an abnormal ortho-static exam?

No

What examination(s) will be abnormal with Postural Orthostatic Tachycardia Syndrome?

Tilt table –
Everything else is often normal

Sudden death, or near sudden death, *precipitated by exercise* is likely to be due to _____?	Anomalous coronary artery/ies (hypertrophic cardiomyopathy and aortic dissection with connective tissue disorder are also possibilities)
In predisposed individuals, being startled can produce a near sudden death episode. What is the mechanism?	Sudden catecholamine surge brings on arrhythmia (loud alarm goes off, hitting the water when diving, car accident, etc.)
How long is too long for the QTc on an EKG?	>0.46 (seconds)
A deaf patient is noted incidentally to have a slightly long QT. What syndrome should you suspect?	Jerveill/Lange-Nielsen (autosomal recessive)
What autosomal dominant long QT syndrome has been especially problematic in females?	Romano-Ward
How do long QT syndromes present?	Incidental finding or syncope, seizure, sudden death
What treatments are used in long QT syndrome?	Pacing, AICDs, β-blockers
If a heart is described as "water-bottle shaped" on x-ray, that is a buzzword for what diagnosis?	Pericarditis/pericardial effusion
You are presented with an EKG that has diffuse S-T changes in no particular pattern, and overall somewhat low voltage. What is your first thought?	Pericarditis
The classic EKG finding for pericardial effusion, which is rarely seen, is _____?	Electrical alternans (A taller and a shorter QRS height alternate across the rhythm strip, due to the heart swinging back and forth in a fluid-filled pericardial sac)

What is the treatment for pericarditis with a small pericardial effusion (not compromising cardiac function)?

NSAIDs

What is the treatment for a significant pericardial effusion that does compromise cardiac function?

Pericardiocentesis

(Surgeon or cardiologist may also place a "pericardial window" to allow continued fluid drainage)

The characteristic chest pain pattern with pericarditis is that it is worse when the patient does what?

Lies down

(Just keep an image in your mind of a pericarditis patient sitting up and leaning forward)

Which two collagen vascular diseases are known for causing pericarditis/pericardial effusions?

Systemic Lupus Erythematosus
   &
Juvenile Idiopathic Arthritis (formerly known as Juvenile Rheumatoid Arthritis)

In addition to collagen vascular diseases, what are two other general causes of pericarditis/pericardial effusion?

1. Infection
2. Post-surgical
(Dressler syndrome – effusion develops 1–2 weeks after cardiac surgery)

Which arrhythmia looks like a "saw tooth" pattern on the EKG?

Atrial flutter

Which arrhythmia looks like a disorganized squiggly line of very low amplitude, with QRSs thrown in?

Atrial fibrillation

A frequent cause of atrial fibrillation in children is _____?

Rheumatic heart disease (although a fib in kids is rare, overall)

How is SVT treated?

1. **Vagal stimulation**
2. **Adenosine**
3. **Synchronized cardioversion**
(if unstable, or not responding to other interventions)

How is ventricular fibrillation treated?

CPR & *defibrillation*!
(not synchronized)

How are stable & unstable ventricular tachycardia treated?

Stable – lidocaine (or amiodarone)
Unstable – Cardioversion
(synchronized, unless there is no pulse)

Can you use a pulse oximeter for the "hyperoxia test?"

No

How is a hyperoxia test done?

ABG on room air, then ABG while child is breathing 100% O$_2$

If the hyperoxia test results show a PaO$_2$>200, what does that mean?

No congenital heart disease (that affects oxygenation, anyway)

If the hyperoxia test results show a PaO$_2$<50, what does that mean?

Restricted pulmonary blood flow, or parallel circuits of blood flow (as in transposition)

(basically, the blood flow is not seeing the oxygen in the lungs)

If the hyperoxia test results show that PaO$_2$ is between 50 and 200, what does that suggest?

A congenital "mixing" lesion is present
(but not causing critical cyanosis)

If postductal saturation is greater than preductal, what congenital anomaly is present?

Transposition of the great arteries!

What is the special name for the results of the test, when the postductal saturation is greater than the preductal?

"Reverse differential" cyanosis

Where is the preductal blood oxygenation measured?

Right hand
(by pulse oximeter)

Where is the postductal blood oxygenation measured?	Either foot (by pulse oximeter)
An enlarged heart with an *increased* stroke volume in a healthy young athlete is likely to be _____?	Athletic heart – do nothing
Are isolated premature atrial contractions worrisome?	Generally, no
Which patients have an increased risk of atrial flutter, if they develop PACs?	<1-year-olds patients on digoxin
What is "sinus arrhythmia?"	Slight variation in the heart rate related to breathing – perfectly normal
In addition to the very recognizable delta wave of Wolf-Parkinson-White, what other EKG abnormality is noted in these patients?	Short P-R interval
If a patient has a long QT syndrome, what family history is usually mentioned?	Sudden death in young family members (Many cases are inherited, although sporadic mutations are now also recognized as a cause, so affected family members are not *always* seen.)
Do all SVTs require treatment?	No – if they are not too fast, and not compromising CV function, they can often be observed
If you are presented with a stable patient in SVT, what is the *first thing to do*?	Get a 12-lead EKG
Should you use verapamil in children?	No – tendency to hypotension/arrest
What electrical conduction abnormality means that most antiarrhythmic medications are contraindicated?	WPW (including digoxin – use procainamide or amiodarone)

If other interventions are not successful to stop an SVT, what electrical solutions can be considered?

Atrial overdrive pacing (pace the heart *faster* than the arrhythmia to "break" the circuit)
& synchronized cardioversion

If an SVT patient is unstable, what is the correct intervention?

Cardioversion (synchronized) *or adenosine if the IV line is already in place*

What relatively common infectious diseases sometimes cause AV block?
    (Name 2 diseases)

Viral myocarditis
    &
Lyme disease

(some zebras, too, such as Chagas disease)

Why is RVH (right ventricular hypertrophy) an *expected* finding in young infants with structurally normal hearts?

Because the RV is the main pumping chamber for the fetus – the thickness normally regresses after birth

(Path is RV to main pulmonary artery, to PDA, to aorta.)

Aortic valve stenosis normally causes *left* ventricular hypertrophy. Why would a neonate with aortic valve stenosis have *right* ventricular hypertrophy?
    (Name 2 reasons)

The RV is the main pumping chamber for the fetus, so it is always (relatively) hypertrophied in neonates
    &
The aortic valve is not part of the circuit until after birth (so no effect)

What is the path for blood circulating through the heart from the RV the fetal period?

RV to main pulmonary artery,

Then to the PDA,

Then to the aorta

What EKG finding do you expect in Tetralogy of Fallot?

Right Ventricular Hypertrophy

(the RV is pushing against a small pulmonic valve, so this makes sense)

If there is an AV canal defect, what will the EKG show?

Left axis deviation (or "superior axis").
(just has to do with the way the electrical system works in that case)

In an older child, CHF can present in what sometimes subtle ways?	Cough Fatigue Poor appetite Poor exercise tolerance
In any child, what physical findings go along with CHF?	Edema Hepatomegaly Jugular venous distention Cardiomegaly Gallop rhythm
What is the usual prophylactic regimen for bacterial endocarditis?	Amoxicillin 1 h before procedure
Which procedures may put the patient at risk for bacterial endocarditis, if she/he has abnormal valves or a murmur?	Oral procedures (including surgery in the area)
Subacute bacterial endocarditis that develops after a tooth extraction is probably due to what organism?	*Strep viridans*
What is the *best test* to confirm bacterial endocarditis?	Blood culture (multiple cultures are often required)
In endocarditis, which type of lesion is painful and usually occurs on the finger and toe pads?	Osler lesions (Remember that an Oslerian history is painful to write up, because it is so complete)
Non-tender red lesions on the hands and feet associated with endocarditis are called _____?	Janeway lesions
Does JIA (Juvenile Idiopathic Arthritis) cause valvular heart disease?	No – it can cause myocarditis/pericarditis
Does rheumatic heart disease cause carditis?	No – only valvular lesions (Carditis is part of rheumatic *fever*)

In acute bacterial endocarditis, what is the usual pathogen?	*Staph aureus*
Does the presence of a murmur affect whether there is an indication for SBE prophylaxis or not?	No
If a patient has had SBE in the past, should she/he always receive prophylaxis in the future?	Yes
If a patient has hypertrophic cardiomyopathy, but no specific valvular lesion, should that patient receive SBE prophylaxis?	No
If a patient has artificial valves or other artificial material as part of their heart valves, should she/he receive SBE prophylaxis?	Yes
If a patient has cyanotic heart disease (not definitively repaired) should she/he receive SBE prophylaxis?	Yes
If a patient has had definitive repair of a cyanotic heart lesion, should SBE prophylaxis still be used?	Yes – In the first 6 months (regardless of how it was repaired) & If residual epithelial defects are known to be present
What about cardiac transplantation patients – do they require SBE prophylaxis for life?	No – Only if valvular lesions are present
What are the buzzwords for innocent murmurs in childhood?	Venous hum Vibratory Musical Carotid bruit
Should an infant with an innocent murmur have any associated physiological findings?	No – if there *any* physiological abnormalities, it's probably not an innocent murmur

If an infant is diagnosed with 3rd-degree heart block, what diagnosis should you suspect for the mother?

Systemic Lupus Erythematosus

(Mom may develop the disorder later, if she doesn't have it now – but some never do)

If a VSD is really large, what unexpected auscultatory exam result might you get?

No murmur – the hole is too big to produce one

What other important auscultatory finding goes with a large VSD?

Single second heart sound (not split), or loud S2

What physical exam finding would go along with a large VSD (not an auscultatory finding)?

Hyperdynamic precordium

(the heart's working really hard to pump the blood, because it keeps sloshing back into the right side)

Ebstein anomaly is associated with maternal use of which prescription medication?

Lithium

VSDs & ASDs are associated with maternal use of what drug of abuse?

Alcohol

Pansystolic (same as holosystolic) murmurs in a child are likely to be due to what three causes?

PDA or venous hum (benign)
   &
VSD
(especially in older children)

Which diastolic-only murmurs are normal findings?

None

Can a 3rd heart sound be normal in children?

Yes
(often heard if the child is lying down)

Can a 4th heart sound be normal in children?

No

Are "harsh" murmurs, or very loud ones, likely to be normal variations?

No
(Greater than 3/6 is not benign – 3/6 rarely)

Do some people have clicks as a normal variant?	Not people with normal hearts – no
Is a cranial bruit likely to be innocent or pathological?	Pathological only
If a patient has "bounding" carotid pulses, and decreased peripheral pulses, what does that suggest?	AV malformation (including cerebral)
Should children with Marfan syndrome participate in athletics?	Not if they have significant dilatation of the aortic root (minimal dilatation is thought to be okay for sports)
What are the most common infectious causes of myocarditis?	Coxsackie A & B viruses (especially Coxsackie B)
What physical findings are noted in myocarditis?	CHF findings, and *no murmur*
If a myocarditis patient has pulsus paradoxus, what would that make you think?	Possible pericardial effusion (causing tamponade)
How do you document a diagnosis of viral myocarditis?	Viral serology & cultures
Most cyanotic congenital heart lesions start with what letter of the alphabet?	"T"
Why would the boards give you a hematocrit, as part of the vignette for congenital heart disease?	Because infants with very low hematocrits, or a lot of fetal hemo-globin, will not show clinical signs of cyanosis until their O₂ level is very low
Children with cyanotic heart disease are at risk for cognitive impairment. What two aspects of their surgical history partly determine their risk for cognitive impairment?	1. Seizure shortly after surgery 2. >75 min on bypass

Cyanosis without respiratory distress suggests what unusual disorder?	Methemoglobinemia
How is methemoglobinemia treated, acutely & in the long term?	Acutely – methylene blue Long term – Remove the triggering chemical (medication, component of well water, etc.)
What is the usual mechanism for an infant or young child to have an episode of methemoglobinemia?	Well water (formula mixed with well water, etc., containing a chemical or heavy metal)
How does a PDA impact the hyperoxia test for congenital heart disease?	It can make them falsely normal, or close to normal
If a newborn presents acutely with a congenital cardiac anomaly, how do they usually present?	Cardiogenic shock or cyanosis
What is the problem in total anomalous pulmonary venous return (TAPVR)?	No oxygenated blood goes to the left side of the heart (unless there is an extra connection)
If there is no "extra" connection to the left side of the heart, what happens to infants with TAPVR?	Not compatible with life
If a full-term newborn is presented in what seems like RDS, what disorder is likely?	TAPVR
Although the right heart is often very active in TAPVR, due to the extra blood flow, what is the overall heart size?	Normal or small
Following surgical correction of TAPVR, left ventricular function can be a bit of a problem. In particular, why is that the case with TAPVR infants?	The LV is (relatively) hypoplastic, due to the structural disorder

How do you expect a TAPVR baby to present, if his/her lesion is compatible with life?

Pulmonary congestion/edema
Cyanosis
Wide split S2
(can also have a short systolic murmur)

What does it mean if TAPVR is "obstructed?"

Blood flow through the returning pulmonary venous vessels is restricted (usually due to passing through the diaphragm) –
so they are "obstructed"

What are the two clinical presentations of TAPVR?

Obstructed and unobstructed

A full-term infant was healthy at birth but becomes cyanotic on the first to second day of life. What is the problem?

The ductus is closing, and this infant has a ductal circulation dependent congenital malformation

Cyanosis, with tachypnea, but no abnormal lung markings, on the first or second day of life suggests _____?

Ductal-dependent circulation with a congenital malformation (the ductus is closing)

If an infant has ductal-dependent circulation, and the ductus is *closing*, how can you treat him/her?

Prostaglandin – it will keep the ductus open

If medication is not successful in keeping the ductus patent, what is another option?

Balloon atrial septostomy by interventional cardiology

How is pulmonary hypertension in a newborn treated?

Inhaled oxygen & nitric oxide, ECMO if needed

Does tricuspid atresia cause cyanosis?

Yes – first of all, it starts with a "T"!!!
Second, if you can't get blood to the RV, you can't get it to the lungs

(at least not without a ductus!)

On a cardiac catheterization, what should the oxygen saturation be in the right side of the heart?

About 70 (%)

What should the oxygen saturation be in the left side of the heart, when measured in a cardiac catheterization?	**About 100 (%)** (like on an ABG, which is also taken from the arterial side of the circulation)
What is the most common cyanotic heart abnormality in children?	**Tetralogy of Fallot**
What is the most common cyanotic heart condition in newborns?	**Transposition of the great arteries**
What are the components of Tetralogy of Fallot?	**P Pulmonary Stenosis** **O Overriding aorta** (overrides the septum) **S Septal Defect (VSD)** **H Hypertrophy – RV**
Do Tetralogy of Fallot babies usually present in the newborn period?	**No – typically it's a 3–5-month-old baby, although some present earlier or later**

What kinds of problems do Tetralogy of Fallot kids have *after* repair?
    (Name 3 problems)
	Arrhythmias
	 Recurrent pulmonary artery obstruction
	    &
	 Syncope

What are the findings of Tetralogy of Fallot? (there are four findings, just as there are four characteristics of the condition)	1. **RV hypertrophy on EKG** 2. **RV heave** 3. **Boot-shaped heart on CXR** 4. **Single S2**
Will the pulmonary vasculature be unusually full, or unusually empty, on CXR with Tetralogy of Fallot?	Empty (decreased) – due to pulmonary stenosis
What is a "Tet spell?"	**An acute episode of hypoxemia in a child with Tetralogy of Fallot**
What causes a Tet spell?	**Acutely increased right to left shunting**

What are the most common triggers for a Tet spell? **(Name 3 triggers)**	• **Crying** (increases pulmonary resistance) • **Warm bath/exercise** (decreases systemic resistance) • **Anemia** (it is not very intuitive that this would cause an acute change in shunting, but it can)
How are Tet spells managed initially?	**Put kid in a squatting position (or knees to chest in an infant!), to shift the pressure back a bit** **(increased peripheral resistance will decrease the R → L shunt)**
What interventions (medications & other sorts) are helpful as short-term follow-up care for a Tet spell?	**Oxygen & Morphine** (decreases right sided pressure) **Phenylephrine & volume expansion** (increased vascular resistance) **Propranolol IV**
What develops abnormally in hypoplastic left heart syndrome?	**Left ventricle** **Aortic valve & Aorta** **Mitral valve**
Is cyanosis evident in infants with hypoplastic left heart syndrome when they are born?	**Usually not**
What is the main problem in hypoplastic left heart syndrome?	**Hypoperfusion** (cyanosis is no picnic, either, but the inability to perfuse is the bigger problem)
Are hypoplastic left heart syndrome babies cyanotic?	**They are often gray, rather than blue** (it's the mix of cyanosis and underperfusion)
Which two congenital heart anomalies have a single S2 sound on auscultation? (There are others, but they are rare!)	**Tetralogy of Fallot** & **Transposition of the Great Vessels**
How can you easily differentiate Tetralogy of Fallot from Transposition of the Great Vessels on CXR?	**Tetralogy of Fallot has *decreased* lung markings** **Transposition has *normal or increased* lung markings**

During what period of life is right ventricular hypertrophy normal?

First few weeks of life

Why is a PDA so important to infants with cyanotic ductal-dependent heart conditions?

Usually because the PDA functions as a replacement pulmonary artery, providing the main blood supply to the lungs!

How does oxygenated & not-oxygenated blood mix, in kids with Transposition of the Great Arteries?

Patent foramen ovale/atrial septal defect
  Or
Ventral septal defect

(Note: Mixing does not occur "via" the PDA – the PDA just helps it along by changing the pressure differential in the atria)

Why is a patent ductus important to increase oxygenation in Transposition of the Great Arteries?

Because the flow it allows increases left atrial pressure, increasing mixing at the atrial level

Are children with Transposition of the Great Arteries "ductal dependent" for oxygenation?

Yes –
unless a large enough atrial communication is there (naturally or created)

If the atrial opening is large enough, the blood will mix anyway, & the extra pressure generated by PDA blood flow is no longer needed

(Pulmonary atresia & Tetralogy of Fallot are also duct dependent)

Are all Tetralogy of Fallot cases "ductal dependent" for oxygenation?

No –
Severe ones often are, though

How can the adequacy of digoxin dosing be effectively monitored in young children?

Check the PR interval

PR interval approaching 200 ms – bordering on 1st-degree heart block – is the goal

If a child has hypertrophic cardiomyopathy, what are some easy ways to test for this while auscultating?

Standing or Valsalva will increase the murmur
(by decreasing the amount of flow through the heart, bringing the ventricular walls closer together)

What special activity limitation is required for children with hypertrophic cardiomyopathy?

No sports or other significant exertion

What is the most common manner in which hypertrophic cardiomyopathy is inherited?

Autosomal dominant

Which part of the heart enlarges in hypertrophic cardiomyopathy?

Ventricular septum
(and left ventricle stiffens)

What is the unusual type of pulse seen in hypertrophic cardiomyopathy?

Double-peaked

How is hypertrophic cardiomyopathy treated?
   (Name 2 medications, 1 device)

Beta-blockers
   &
Calcium channel blockers
   &
AICDs (implanted defibrillator)

What will you see on EKG in hypertrophic cardiomyopathy?

Left ventricular hypertrophy & left axis deviation

If hypertrophic cardiomyopathy patients have symptoms, what are the typical symptoms?

Chest pain with exertion
Dyspnea
Syncope

What does it mean if a congenital heart abnormality is "duct dependent?"

The ductus is the main source allowing oxygenated blood to get to either the body or lungs

Which congenital cardiac problems are the classic "ductal-dependent" lesions seen on board examinations?

Transposition
Tetralogy of Fallot
Pulmonary Atresia

Some ductal-dependent heart lesions allow increased blood flow to the lungs. Others allow increased blood flow to where?

The systemic circulation!

What are the main heart-related conditions that compromise systemic blood flow and are helped by a PDA?
 (Name 3 conditions)

Critical aortic stenosis
Severe aortic coarctation
& Interrupted aortic arch

In which ductal-dependent heart conditions is the PDA needed to increase pulmonary blood flow?

Tetralogy of Fallot
Pulmonary artery atresia
Tricuspid atresia

(Specifically, Tetralogy of Fallot with significant pulmonary atresia & Pulmonary atresia with intact intraventricular septum – PA/IVS)

In truncus arteriosus, what ventricular abnormality is nearly always present?

Large VSD

Why does TAPVR have a wide, fixed, split S2?

An ASD allows blood to the left side of the heart

What are the three types of TAPVR?

Pulmonary veins return to:
1. Superior vena cava
2. Right atrium
3. Inferior vena cava/hepatic or portal veins

Which type of TAPVR is usually obstructed?

The one that enters the venous system low, by the liver, because the vessels pass through the diaphragm. (Pressure from the diaphragm causes some obstruction.)

What special problem will TAPVR patients with obstruction usually have?

Pulmonary hypertension, due to difficulty emptying the pulmonary vasculature

Is transposition of the great vessels a survivable abnormality?

Only if another connection to the left side of the circulation exists (such as a PFO, ASD, or VSD)

Chapter 2
Pulmonology: The Lungs, Oxygen, and Perfusion

Arteries in the pulmonary vasculature *constrict* if the air in the alveoli near them doesn't have the expected amount of oxygen (approximately 21 % or greater at sea level). Substances that make this response even more pronounced are:

Dopamine
Propranolol
Almitrine (a ventilatory stimulant)
Acidosis

Substances or situations that blunt this "hypoxic lung response" by the pulmonary arterial system include:

Beta agonists
Calcium channel blockers
Anesthetics
Prostaglandins
Vasodilators (in general)
High cardiac output (pushes more blood into the constricted areas)
Alkalosis

If one of these "blunting" circumstances is present, and your patient has a mismatch between the ventilation and perfusion of the lung, *the mismatch will actually worsen*! This makes sense because areas that are *not* well ventilated will be well perfused.

Remember that "V" stands for "ventilation" when oxygenation is being discussed, while "Q" stands for "perfusion." There must be a story as to how the letter "Q" was selected, but I haven't heard it.

Also remember that, throughout the normal lung, there are a variety of V:Q ratios. The top of the lung ordinarily receives more ventilation than it should for its amount of blood flow, because gravity has a big effect on the blood flow in the lung.

The bottom of the lung, on the other hand, is overperfused, and doesn't have great ventilation. Think of it as gravity making it hard to lift and open the bottom

C.M. Houser, *Pediatric Cardiology and Pulmonology: A Practically Painless Review*,
DOI 10.1007/978-1-4614-9481-2_2, © Springer Science+Business Media New York 2014

part of the lung, so it's not very well ventilated, yet the blood likes to pool there, because it's at the bottom of the lung.

Blood samples that we obtain reflect the "average" of all of the V:Q relationships throughout the lung.

Neonates and Normal Oxygen Tension

Interestingly, normal neonates close off significant portions of their lung during ordinary exhalation (due to low chest wall compliance, mainly). This means that their PaO_2 (arterial partial pressure of oxygen) is normally significantly lower than you would expect in an adult or an older child.

The Alveolar Gas Equation and the A–a Gradient

The alveolar gas equation allows us to calculate how much oxygen is in the alveoli. We need to do this to anticipate how much oxygen should be circulating in the blood. The amount of the oxygen in the alveoli is expressed as the partial pressure of oxygen in the alveoli (in the equations, alveolar values have a capital "A").

The partial pressure of oxygen in the alveoli is always a little less than the partial pressure of oxygen in the air inspired. Why is that?

The partial pressure of oxygen must be *less* in the alveoli than in the air inspired because alveolar oxygen is mixed with both the carbon dioxide leaving the blood via the alveolar capillary and diffusing into the alveolus, and because there is always some water vapor doing the same thing. The alveolar gas equation therefore includes a factor for the partial pressure of the water vapor and a factor for the carbon dioxide the body is releasing into the alveolus. The alveolar partial pressure of oxygen usually works out to be 100, at sea level.

The Alveolar Gas Equation

$$PAO_2 = (\text{fraction } O_2 \text{ inspired})(\text{barometric P - water vapor P}) - PaCO_2 / 0.8$$

Room air inspired O_2 fraction $= 0.21$ (this may be more if you are giving O_2).
Barometric pressure $-$ water vapor pressure $= 760 - 47 = 713$.
The whole first term is usually, therefore, $713(0.21)$, which equals 150.

The arterial pressure of CO_2 is taken from the ABG measurement of CO_2. It is divided by 0.8 as a correction factor, because the body produces a little less CO_2 than it consumes O_2.

The whole equation equals about 100, if a healthy patient is breathing room air at about sea level.

The A–a Gradient

We expect the partial pressure of oxygen in the blood to be at a certain level for any given level of oxygen in the alveolar air. There are a few factors in the body's use of oxygen that make the two oxygen tensions slightly different, but they do have a predictable relationship:

$$PAO_2 - PaO_2 = A - aO_2 \text{ gradient}$$

In English, the alveolar partial pressure of oxygen – the arterial partial pressure of oxygen = the gradient, or the difference, between them. *The normal gradient in a healthy young adult is around 10, and in children it can be less than 10.*

Non-pulmonary reasons that the A–a gap can widen, or increase, include advancing age (the elderly), obesity, fasting, lying supine for an extended period, and vigorous exercise.

Hypoxemia

How does it happen?

1. Alveolar hypoventilation – If the patient doesn't breathe in enough oxygen, the patient becomes hypoxic/hypoxemic (for example, due to CNS depression or muscular weakness).
2. Diffusion impairment – If the patient breathes in enough oxygen, but the oxygen can't easily cross the alveolar membrane (due to thickening, or due to something coating or covering the membrane), then the patient may become hypoxemic.
3. Intrapulmonary shunting – If too much blood is shunted to the left side of the heart without being properly ventilated in the alveoli, then the patient may become hypoxic. This can occur due to structural problems in the vasculature and also due to areas of collapsed or fluid-filled alveoli.
4. V:Q mismatch – If too much blood is sent to poorly ventilated areas of the lung (such as the bottom of the lung or an area with a blocked bronchus), V:Q mismatch will occur. If the mismatch is significant enough, the patient will become hypoxic.

Similarly, if areas of lung are being ventilated, but not very well perfused, as is the case with a pulmonary embolus, then the patient may become hypoxic.

Chapter 3
General Pulmonary Question and Answer Items

What is the most common chronic pediatric disorder?	Asthma
Is the incidence & prevalence of asthma been increasing or decreasing?	**Both increasing**
Is the morbidity & mortality from asthma increasing or decreasing?	**Both increasing** (some studies show that M&M is leveling out, but for the boards use increasing)
Which children are most likely to experience serious morbidity & mortality from asthma? (demographic factors)	• Poor children • Inner-city children • African-American
What type of asthma puts children at highest risk of death from an acute asthma episode?	Mild asthma (>80 % of deaths were in children with mild asthma histories)
What proportion of children who have asthma should be on chronic medication for the disorder?	¾
What is the relationship between household pets and asthma?	*More pets = less asthma risk* (*it's best to have at least two – it has to do with a bacterial endotoxin on dogs & cats*)

C.M. Houser, *Pediatric Cardiology and Pulmonology: A Practically Painless Review*,
DOI 10.1007/978-1-4614-9481-2_3, © Springer Science+Business Media New York 2014

What is the "hygiene hypothesis" for the etiology of asthma?

Lack of microbial exposure in developed countries prevents a normal shift from fetal Type 2 Helper T-Cell dominance to Type 1 Helper T-Cell dominance

Type 2 Helper T's promote allergy

What is the prevalence of asthma in developing countries?

<2 %

What is the role of obesity in asthma?

Seems to be pro-inflammatory

If you have two dogs in the household, how much lower is your kid's risk of developing asthma, compared to kids with no pets?

About 18 % on the average

PFTs can't be done properly on very young children. How is asthma diagnosed in these very young children, if they seem to have symptoms?

**Clinically –
Repeated episodes of wheezing, coughing, retractions/use of accessory muscles, tachypnea without other explanation
     &
Response to typical asthma medications**

Which PFTs should be used in older children to document asthma?

**FEV$_1$
     &
FEV$_1$/FVC**

Why is it important to begin appropriate treatment of asthma, for children requiring long-term medication, as soon as possible?

Because permanent damage (airway remodeling) occurs in the first few years

After permanent changes occur in the lung of an asthma patient, can you still improve pulmonary symptoms?

Yes – symptoms will improve but lung function will not return to normal

What is the most important part of asthma medication treatment – inhaled steroids or inhaled beta-agonists?

Steroids – inflammation seems to be the main issue

Do children with mild asthma develop structural changes in the lung?

Yes – thickening of basement membranes

"Transient wheezing" that does not develop into asthma usually occurs in what setting?

Young children with viral illnesses

Which kids are at biggest risk for "transient wheezing" episodes?

- Boys
- h/o low birth weight
- Maternal smoking during & after pregnancy

What anatomic difference has been observed in children with transient wheezing?

Smaller than average airways and lungs

If a child wheezes before age 3, what major risk criteria indicate a high risk of chronic asthma?

- **Parental asthma**
- **Eczema**
- **Sensitivity to inhaled allergens**

If a child wheezes before age 3, what minor risk criteria indicate a high risk of chronic asthma (if the child has two of the risk criteria)?

- Wheezing without URI
- Food sensitivities
- Eosinophilia ≥ 4 %

The risk factors just mentioned are the criteria for what index, developed by following 1,000 children to identify likely risk factors for asthma after age 5?

The Asthma Predictive Index

Which children does the index just mentioned apply to?

Children <3 years old with four or more episodes of wheezing over a 1-year period

(The Asthma Predictive Index)

What is the expected percentage of normal FEV_1 for children with moderate persistent asthma?

60–80 %

(severe asthma is <60 %, naturally)

What is the expected percentage of predicted FEV_1 for children with mild forms of asthma (persistent & intermittent)?

≥ 80 %

Many children "grow out of" asthma. When does that usually happen?	**At puberty**
If a child's asthma is not controlled when he or she reaches the critical age for "growing out of" asthma, is it likely to go away?	**No**
If a child with asthma is obese when he/she reaches puberty, is the asthma likely to remit?	**Less likely**
In addition to obesity and poor control of asthma, what other factors are associated with continuing asthma through adolescence?	Sinusitis & environmental allergies not under good control at puberty
Which paromyxovirus causes an RSV-like infection in late winter and early spring?	Human metapneumovirus
Which cardiac problem often presents like RSV, especially in very young infants & children?	Congestive heart failure
An infant is brought in for an apnea. A coughing adolescent sibling accompanies mom and baby. What are these two clues supposed to tell you?	**That the infant caught pertussis from the adolescent (could also be a coughing mom) –** *Apnea – or seizure – is a fairly common pertussis presentation for infants*
What is a common, and worrisome, presentation for pertussis in infants?	**Apnea!**
What is the mortality for infants presenting with apnea due to pertussis?	50 %
Pertussis is most severe in which age group?	**Infants**
Bilateral empyemas and a scarlatiniform rash strongly suggest what diagnosis?	Group A strep pneumonia

A pneumonia that begins within hours of birth, and has a fulminant course, is likely due to what organism?	**Grp B strep**
If you are treating a bacterial pneumonia in a child between a month of age and 10 years, what organisms must you cover?	*Staph aureus & Strep pneumo*
For patients older than 10 years, which organisms will you mainly cover, if you believe the patient has a bacterial pneumonia?	*Strep pneumo &* atypicals
What is the most common (immediate) cause of cardiac arrest in kids?	**Respiratory failure**
In infants, a blocked nose can cause respiratory distress. In older patients, how much of the total airway resistance is determined by the nose?	50 % (!)
How much of the total airway resistance comes from the peripheral airways in a child? Why is this important?	• 50 % (vs. 20 % in an adult) • A little edema in the airways can cause a big problem
Generally speaking, what ABG values indicate that your patient is in respiratory failure?	$pH < 7.3$ PaO_2 and $PaCO_2$ of about 50 each
What kind of a cardiac shunt produces cyanosis?	**Right to left (bypasses the lungs)**
Asthma can increase CO_2 for a variety of reasons. What are the main two?	1. Lack of ventilation when the episode is very bad 2. High intrathoracic pressure squishes the alveolar capillaries, increasing the effective dead space
If the board wants to tell you that a patient is hypoxemic, what are they likely to put in the vignette?	**Change in level of consciousness**

If the board wants to tell you that a patient is hypercarbic, what are they likely to put in the vignette?	**Change in level of consciousness**
If the board wants to tell you that there is an airway obstruction issue, what are they likely to put in the vignette?	**Stridor**
If a patient is described with gray skin coloration and tachycardia, what is the vignette usually trying to tell you?	**Patient is hypoxic**
What do patients with pulmonary hypertension, cor pulmonale, and polycythemia all have in common, in terms of respiratory function?	Chronic respiratory inadequacy/ insufficiency
If a patient lives with chronic respiratory insufficiency, what must you be careful of when treating them with oxygen?	**Suppression of respiratory drive if too much oxygen is given**
How can a respiratory drive be oxygen dependent? I thought it was based on carbon dioxide levels?	Normally, it is based on CO_2 level – with chronic CO_2 retention, though, it switches to O_2
When a boards question lists "Circulation, Airway, Breathing" as one of the answer choices, what should that mean to you?	**It is almost always the right answer!**
If a patient has a respiratory *acidosis*, what <u>must</u> the CO_2 on the ABG show?	**High CO_2** (Just think of CO_2 as acid)
If a patient has a respiratory *alkalosis*, what <u>must</u> the CO_2 on the ABG show?	**Low CO_2**
In a metabolic *alkalosis*, what <u>must</u> be on the ABG?	**High bicarb**

In a metabolic *acidosis*, what <u>must</u> be on the ABG?	Low bicarb
Which pediatric patients are likely to have a metabolic alkalosis?	Those on chronic diuretics, such as BPD patients
Which pediatric patient group is most likely to develop a metabolic acidosis?	Shock (any of the types) or toxin ingestion
When do you see respiratory alkalosis?	Most often, with simple hyperventilation – Also seen with ↑ ICP and encephalopathies, early portion of asthma exacerbation, and salicylate overdose
If you have a patient with acidosis and a low bicarb, which type of metabolic derangement is that?	Metabolic acidosis
If you have a patient with acidosis and a high CO_2, which type of metabolic derangement is that?	Respiratory acidosis
If bicarb is the base that's supposed to take care of (buffer) any extra acid in the body, what do you think will happen to the bicarb level, if the body acids increase?	It should go up to take care of (buffer) the acid (it takes a little while to change the bicarb level, though)
If you have a patient with acidosis and a high CO_2, who also has a high bicarb, what does that mean then?	Partially compensated respiratory acidosis (If it's acidosis with high CO_2, it's still respiratory acidosis – the bicarb went up to *try* to fix the problem. That's why it's partially compensated.)
If CO_2 is acid for the body, what do you think will happen to the CO_2 level if the body gets alkalotic?	It will go up, to try to take care of (buffer) the excess of base/bicarb (this process happens pretty quickly, because it mainly depends on how fast or slow we're breathing)

If you have a patient with alkalosis, and a high bicarb, who also has a high CO_2, what does that mean then?

Partially compensated metabolic alkalosis

(If it's alkalosis with a high bicarb, it's still metabolic alkalosis – the CO_2 went up to *try* to fix the problem. That's why it's partially compensated.)

What is the trend for morbidity and mortality from asthma?

Both increasing

What is the probability that a child will have problems with recurrent wheezing, if the child develops RSV bronchiolitis in the first 3 years of life?

50 %
(may not become asthma, necessarily)

If a patient is having an asthma exacerbation, and the wheezes eventually disappear so that the chest is much quieter, what should you conclude?

Two possibilities –
Either the patient has improved, *or the patient is worse*
(not moving enough air to produce a wheeze)

Early in an asthma exacerbation, what kind of blood gas changes do you expect?

Low CO_2 (due to rapid breathing) & sometimes low O_2

What is the name for the metabolic derangement early in an asthma episode?

Respiratory alkalosis

With impending respiratory failure, what happens to the blood gas values?

CO_2 goes up (poor ventilation) and O_2 goes down

What sort of metabolic derangement do you expect late in a bad asthma exacerbation?

Respiratory acidosis (very little compensation, because the kidney can't adjust the bicarb so quickly)

How can you tell that an asthma patient is heading for respiratory failure, by the way he/she is speaking?

Can't speak or can't speak more than a few words at a time

When should you worry about cyanosis in an asthma patient?

If it's central
(not really a good thing, though, in any part of the patient!)

If you see oral/perioral cyanosis, is that considered to be central cyanosis?

No

If an asthma patient is heading for respiratory failure, what hint can you get from their body positioning?

Won't lie down
(not very specific, though – most patients with a significant asthma exacerbation are anxious, and anxious people don't like to lie down)

Patients with impending respiratory failure often have what skin finding, in addition to cyanosis?

Diaphoresis (especially if the patient is conscious)

What three sorts of risk factors determine a patient's risk for a fatal asthma exacerbation?

1. Medical
2. Psychosocial
3. Ethnicity

How do you know that a child is at increased risk for a *fatal* asthma attack, based on ethnicity?

Non-whites are at greater risk

What characteristics of previous asthma attacks mean that your patient is at increased risk for a *fatal* exacerbation?

1. Rapid decline or severe compromise
2. Respiratory failure
3. Seizure
4. Loss of consciousness

Most of the psychosocial factors that impact a patient's risk for a fatal asthma exacerbation have to do with how likely they are to follow their asthma regimen. What are they?

1. Psychiatric disorder (including depression)
2. Dysfunctional family
3. Denial of disease with (direct) noncompliance

There is a final psychosocial factor that impacts risk for fatal asthma attacks. It is really more of a demographic characteristic. What is it?

Resides in the inner city

Which cardiovascular finding is wildly popular on boards exams, rarely performed in real life, and a sign of impending respiratory failure in an asthmatic?

Pulsus paradoxus

For those of you who don't measure it on a daily basis, what is pulsus paradoxus?	**When the difference between the systolic BP in inspiration vs. expiration is more than 10 mmHg (it's normally <5 mmHg)**
Why does pulsus paradoxus happen?	The variation in systolic BP is due to the change in intrathoracic pressure – it drops with inspiration. That reduces the systolic blood pressure a little
Pulsus paradoxus seems like a mainly cardiovascular thing. Why is it affected by a pulmonary problem like asthma?	If intrathoracic pressure drops *a whole lot* due to making a huge inspiratory effort, the systolic BP is lowered that much further
Can't pulsus paradoxus happen with cardiac problems, too?	Yes – for example, pericardial tamponades are usually worsened by inspiration, lowering cardiac output, and reducing the systolic BP (but the mechanism is different than in asthma)
Should you base your decision to intubate a patient on lab values or on clinical impression?	**Clinical impression**
Why should you be careful to avoid overhydration in patients with chronic lung disease?	**Tendency to SIADH (could make the extra fluid very hard to get rid of)**
Do you need to worry about SIADH in your asthma patients?	Yes
Do you need to worry about suppressing the ventilatory drive when you give O_2 to asthma patients?	No (they don't have chronic hypercarbia, so their drive should still be CO_2 dependent)
What type of peak expiratory flow suggests that an asthma patient can be discharged to home?	**≥70 % of expected peak flow**

After you've treated an asthmatic patient, what level of peak expiratory flow indicates that he/she needs to be admitted to the PICU?

<50 %

If your asthmatic patient's response to treatment is between 50 and 70 %, what disposition is recommended?

Admit to floor

Should you routinely give antibiotics to asthma patients who develop an exacerbation in response to a respiratory infection?

No – most of the infectious triggers are viral

If you need to give a systemic beta-agonist for asthma, what is the preferred agent?

Terbutaline

When is it reasonable to give a systemic beta-agonist?

Response to inhaled treatment is not adequate

Why do beta-agonists improve asthma?

Stimulate the Beta-2 receptors on the smooth muscle (increasing cAMP) which relaxes the smooth muscle

Which is more effective for children with a severe asthma exacerbation, continuous or intermittent nebulization?

Continuous
(it may be a more cost-effective way to deliver nebulization for asthma, in general, also)

Should inhaled ipratropium bromide (Atrovent®) be used for children with asthma exacerbations?

Yes! Every time.

(Especially beneficial for the worst exacerbations)

If an asthma patient is acidotic, should he/she be intubated?

Not automatically – evaluate clinically

There are three absolute indications to intubate an asthmatic. What are they?

1. **Arrest (I think you know that)**
2. **Severe hypoxia**
3. **Rapid deterioration in mental state**

A lot of doctors feel happier with a controlled airway. What are the "downsides" to intubating asthmatics? (List 1 mechanical problem, 1 correlation, 2 ventilation issues)	1. **Sticking the laryngoscope in worsens bronchospasm** 2. **>50 % of morbidity/mortality happens during and immediately after intubation** 3. **Ventilation increases the risk of hypotension** 4. **Ventilation increases the risk of barotrauma**
Why would you want to consider using ketamine when intubating an asthma patient?	Relaxes bronchoconstriction
Why would you want to consider using a cuffed tube after intubating an asthmatic?	Improves ability to ventilate
Is it a good idea to intubate an asthma patient without neuromuscular blockade?	No – Big increases in pleural pressure and increased bronchoconstriction
You have just finished intubating an asthmatic patient, and now the patient has suddenly become hypotensive. What is the best initial management of the hypotension?	**Support pressure with fluid – not pressors** **(also consider whether intrathoracic pressure is too high due to a tension pneumo or not allowing enough time for expiration)**
Are secretions a worry after you've intubated an asthma patient?	**Yes – can obstruct the tube, and are another cause of hypotension post-intubation**
If you set the ventilator to allow for a long expiratory phase, your patient will often continue to be hypercarbic while ventilated. What should you do about this?	Usually nothing – it's called permissive hypercapnia, and is okay as long as the pH and oxygen level are alright
If you are seeing a near-drowning patient in the ER, and they look fine and have a good chest x-ray, is it safe to discharge them home?	**No –** **ARDS often develops hours after the incident. Best to observe in a moni-tored setting for first 24 h**

What is the main problem for the patient with ARDS?	**Not enough oxygen** **(hard to find a way to get O_2 into the blood stream)**
The best way to match ventilation and perfusion in (ventilated) patients with cardiogenic pulmonary edema is _____?	**PEEP** **(Positive End Expiratory Pressure)**
An infant is admitted to the hospital with meningococcemia. She was resuscitated successfully and is receiving IV antibiotics. Twelve hours after admission she becomes tachypneic and hypoxemic. What will her x-ray most likely show?	**Diffuse reticular infiltrate** **(ARDS s/p fluid resuscitation in an ill patient)**
Upper airway obstruction typically produces what symptom?	**Stridor**
What are the three typical signs of lower airway obstruction or constriction?	1. **Cough** 2. **Wheeze** 3. **Prolonged expiratory phase (earliest sign)**
What are normal adult arterial blood gas (ABG) values? ($pH/PaO_2/PaCO_2$)	**7.4/100/40**
At what age should children's blood gases look approximately the same as those of adults?	7 years
The younger the child, the more the ABG differs from adult values. In what three ways is the ABG of a child normally different from that of an adult?	1. O_2 is *lower* 2. CO_2 is *lower* 3. Bicarb is *lower*
What is a normal PaO_2 for children <24 months old?	About 90
What is a normal $PaCO_2$ for children <24 months old?	About 34

The bicarb (HCO_3^-) in an ABG *is calculated*, not measured. What bicarb values are normal for adults vs. children younger than 2 years?

Adult 24

Older infant/toddler 20

At birth, ABGs are wildly different from those of older children. What is a typical birth ABG? ($pH/PaO_2/PaCO_2/HCO_3^-$)

7.27/60/55/19

(*These are not typos! Newborns really have these scary ABG values.*)

Neonates >24 h old have an ABG between that of the birth ABG and toddler ABG. What are the typical values?

7.37/70/33/20

Can a VBG (venous blood gas) be used to evaluate pH if an arterial sample is not available?

Yes –
Venous blood may have a slightly lower pH, but it's very similar

In most children with respiratory problems, how high is your oxygen saturation goal?

>95 %

The mainstay of treatment for reactive airway disease exacerbations is what medication (and dose)?

Nebulized albuterol

(*0.1 mg/kg/dose – just FYI*)

In moderate to severe reactive airway disease (RAD) exacerbations, what other nebulized medication is helpful, in additional to albuterol?

Ipratropium bromide (Atrovent®)
(*0.25–0.5 mg FYI*)

If an RAD patient ordinarily takes steroids, and presents to you with an exacerbation, what medication is definitely indicated?

Oral or IV/IM steroids –
2 mg/kg loading dose

Are parenteral steroids "proven" to have a greater or more rapid effect on RAD exacerbations than oral steroids?

No –
Not for mild to moderate exacerbations

(If exacerbation is *severe*, give IV or IM)

In a severe RAD exacerbation, or if a patient cannot take nebulizer treatments, what other medications may provide rapid relief?
  (Name 2 medications)

1. Epinephrine SQ (0.01 cc/kg of 1:1,000 – maximum dose 0.3 cc's)
2. Terbutaline 0.01 mg/kg SQ (maximum dose 0.4 cc's per dose)

If you are treating RAD with epinephrine or terbutaline, how many times may you repeat the dose?	Three times total, 15 min apart
If an RAD patient does not have significant improvement with the first albuterol treatment, what medication should be added?	Steroids (even if the patient does not take them regularly)
For severe RAD episodes, responsive to terbutaline given SQ, what medication should be started?	Terbutaline infusion, of course!
In addition to epinephrine, steroids, and terbutaline, what other injectable medication may aid in relaxing the smooth muscle of the pulmonary tree?	Magnesium sulfate
If available, what special gas mixture can be used to decrease the work of breathing in either upper airway obstruction or RAD?	Heliox (helium/oxygen mix – studies are mixed as to whether it helps)
When should heliox definitely *not* be used?	When the patient is severely hypoxic – (It is mixed with helium so the FiO_2 is less than a rebreather mask or similar device)
In addition to treatment with medications, asthma patients need to identify triggers for their exacerbations. What are four common ones?	1. Cold 2. Exertion 3. Upper respiratory infections 4. Irritants (pollen, dander, smoke, etc.)
How is childhood asthma categorized? **(4)**	1. **Mild intermittent** 2. **Mild persistent (<1 episode per day, but more than 2 per week)** 3. **Moderate persistent** 4. **Severe persistent**
What is the only level of chronic asthma that can be treated without daily medication?	**Mild intermittent**

In general, what is the guiding principle in RAD treatment?

Be aggressive –
(When you have gained good control of the problem, you can gradually decrease treatment as tolerated)

What is the most common cause of bronchiolitis?

RSV
(other viruses & mycoplasma also cause it)

What percentage of infants with bronchiolitis will have RAD later?

50 %

(It often resolves after age 3)

What age group is mainly affected by bronchiolitis?

<12 months
        &
especially <3 months

How is RSV spread?
  (Name 2 mechanisms)

1. **Mainly direct secretion contact**
2. **Droplets**

Do bronchiolitis patients usually have rhinorrhea & thick nasal secretions?

Yes
(That's how it spreads so easily via secretions)

What are two important environmental or demographic risk factors for the development of bronchiolitis?

1. Low socioeconomic status (due to crowding, more frequent delay in immunizations, etc.)

2. Exposure to smoke – especially cigarette smoke

Rapid viral test are available for diagnosis of RSV. If negative, what follow-up test should be sent?

Nasopharyngeal culture

Bronchiolitis is an annoying but benign disease for most infants. In very general terms, which patients are likely to have serious complications?

Those with comorbidities (including prematurity)

In addition to viral tests, what labs or diagnostics should you order for a bronchiolitis patient?
  (Name 4)

1. CBC with differential
2. Pulse ox
3. ABG (depending on severity of illness)
4. Chest x-ray

What complications are seen in bronchiolitis?	1. **Pneumonia** 2. **Apnea** 3. **Respiratory distress & failure** 4. **Pneumothorax (with coughing or mechanical ventilation)**
Which airways are affected in bronchiolitis?	Bronchioles, silly! (They're the small airways before the alveolar sacs)
Why do the airways become swollen in bronchiolitis?	The virus attacks the respiratory epithelium yielding inflammation
Why do the small airways become obstructed in bronchiolitis?	Normal respiratory epithelium dies – The replacement cells do not initially have cilia (so secretions don't move!)
Why might an infant with bronchiolitis seem to have hepato-splenomegaly?	The hyperinflated lungs move these organs down
A history of apnea, cyanosis, or respiratory distress in an infant with bronchiolitis suggests what complication is likely?	Impending respiratory failure
Do patients with bronchiolitis usually have a fever?	Yes – Low grade
When might theophylline be useful in bronchiolitis?	Apneic patients – It stimulates the respiratory drive
What are the typical findings of bronchiolitis on chest x-ray? (Name 3)	1. Hyperinflation 2. Atelectasis 3. Diffuse interstitial infiltrates
Do infants with bronchiolitis improve when treated with aerosolized β-adrenergic agents? (in other words, albuterol)	Sometimes (Infants with a personal or family history of wheezing are most likely to benefit)

In addition to supportive care and β-adrenergic agents, are antibiotics, steroids, or antiviral agents helpful in the treatment of RSV bronchiolitis?	Antibiotics – no Steroids – probably not Antivirals – no (Aerosolized ribavirin no longer considered helpful for the most severely ill infants as of 2004)
Although the use of ribavirin is controversial in RSV treatment, what three beneficial effects has it been shown to have?	1. Improved O_2 saturation 2. Shortened illness duration 3. Shortened period of viral shedding
If a child with RSV requires mechanical ventilation, weaning & extubation is often difficult. Why?	Copious secretions & atelectasis
What are typical signs of impending respiratory failure? (Name 4 signs)	1. $\downarrow O_2$ 2. $\uparrow CO_2$ 3. Retractions 4. Lethargy (or sometimes agitation)
Does RSV bronchiolitis require isolation?	If admitted, yes (Meaning don't mix them with non-RSV patients)
If a child has recovered from RSV bronchiolitis, can they become reinfected?	Yes – Even in the same season!
How long is the typical course of RSV?	Usually improves in <5 days, but cough may persist for *weeks*
Chlamydial organisms can cause pneumonia in children & adults – which chlamydial organism affects neonates and which affects older children/adults?	Neonates/infants – Chlamydia trachomatis Children/adults – Chlamydia pneumoniae
I have a nagging feeling there's another sort of chlamydia that causes pneumonia. Is there?	Yes, Chlamydia psittaci – Comes from birds Much less common

What triad of symptoms goes with croup?	**Barking cough** **Stridor** **Hoarseness** (*All are due to subglottic stenosis*)
What is the other (more official) name for croup?	Laryngotracheobronchitis Mnemonic: LTB stands for Laryngo-Tracheo-Bronchitis or Long-Term Bark!
In general terms, what causes croup?	Many viruses (mainly parainfluenza, but also RSV, adenovirus, etc.)
What is spasmodic croup?	Sudden onset of inspiratory stridor for a several-hour period – Recurs for several days – Usually happens at night
What is the typical age for croup?	6 months–36 months (most common between 1 and 2 years)
Is croup more common in males or females?	Males (3:2)
What is the natural course of croup?	Complete recovery
What are the main complications of croup? (Name 3 complications)	1. Respiratory failure (rare) 2. Airway obstruction 3. *Hypoxia*
Why does airway obstruction sometimes develop in croup infection?	*First*, the immune response creates surplus sections, *then* – It causes erythema & edema of cords and upper airway
Why are subglottic areas most affected by the swelling of croup?	The cricoid cartilage sits there, and it limits the diameter of the airway
If a child seems to have croup, but doesn't have a fever, and the onset of symptoms was while awake & playing – what other diagnosis should be considered?	**Foreign body aspiration**

If you suspect a diagnosis of croup, what x-rays might you want?
(Name 2)

Chest x-ray
(rule-out foreign body, pneumonia)
&
AP & lateral soft tissue neck x-rays
(rule-out epiglottitis, pharyngeal abscess)

What are the typical x-ray findings of croup?
(Name 2 findings)

"Steeple sign"
(on AP neck)
&
Chest x-ray may show atelectasis

What is the typical duration of croup infections?

3–5 days

Why should you wait at least 3–4 h after treatment with racemic epinephrine before discharging a croup patient?

Croup patients often have a rebound as much as 2 h after the treatment

How can croup be treated
(if treatment is necessary)?
(Name 3 treatments)

1. Cool, humified air
2. Nebulized racemic epinephrine
   (0.5 mL of 2.25 %)
3. Dexamethasone IM

If a croup patient is thought to have impending respiratory failure, what is the *next step* in management?

Intubation *in the OR*

(do not delay for x-ray or other tests)

When is racemic epinephrine indicated for croup?
(Name 2)

Extreme respiratory distress
   Or
Minimal response to humidified air

What five factors are evaluated in the croup severity score?

1. Inspiratory stridor
2. Retractions
3. Air entry (how much it is decreased)
4. Cyanosis
5. Level of consciousness

If a child suffers from recurrent croup, what should be investigated?

1. Anatomic abnormalities
2. Congenital anomalies
3. GE reflux

Why is IM dexamethasone preferred to oral prednisone in croup treatment? (Name 4 reasons)	1. Efficacy of oral steroid is not clear 2. Croup patients often have poor oral intake 3. Less GI distress 4. Longer half-life (about 48 h vs. 24 h)
What is the most common cause of cor pulmonale?	Parenchymal lung disease (sometimes other types of lung disease also cause it)
What causes cor pulmonale?	Chronic hypoxia → Pulmonary vasoconstriction and pulmonary hypertension → High RV afterload
When does cor pulmonale usually start?	In teens of 20s – *Especially with pregnancy* (can be found at any age, though)
Why does the right ventricle fail in cor pulmonale?	The afterload of the pulmonary vasculature is too much for it
What are the typical complications of cor pulmonale? (Name 3 complications)	1. Anemia or polycythemia (can go either way) 2. RV failure 3. Sudden death
Why are cor pulmonale patients at risk for sudden death?	They cannot augment cardiac output with exercise
What physical findings are expected in cor pulmonale? (4 – do not give auscultation findings)	1. Parasternal heave 2. JVD/hepatomegaly/peripheral edema 3. Tachycardia 4. Cyanosis
What do cor pulmonale patients usually complain of? (Name 5 complaints)	Fatigue Syncope Palpitations Chest pain Poor exercise tolerance
How can upper airway disease cause cor pulmonale?	The hypoxia leads to pulmonary vasoconstriction

Why do newborn infants have less trouble with RV failure secondary to pulmonary hypertension?

Both ventricles have a similar structure at birth (so the RV is stronger then than it will be later)

If the right ventricle is strong enough to "stand up" to the pressure of pulmonary hypertension, why do neonates develop heart failure with cor pulmonale?

Secondary to the hypoxemia & acidosis of the condition

Is nocturnal O_2 useful for cor pulmonale patients, in general?

No –
But it may delay progression in individuals with obstructive sleep hypoxia producing cor pulmonale

What diagnostic procedure is indicated for *all* cor pulmonale patients?

Cardiac catheterization

What are the main invasive measurements needed in cardiac catheterization for cor pulmonale?

Pulmonary artery pressure
   &
Reaction of pulmonary vasculature to oxygen & various medications

What are the two most common causes of eosinophilic pneumonia?

1. Drug reactions (therapeutic or recreational drugs)
2. Parasites

What proportion of eosinophilic pneumonias has no known etiology?

1/3

How is eosinophilic pneumonia diagnosed?
   (Name 3)

1. Infiltrates + peripheral eosinophilia
2. Infiltrates + >5 % eosinophils in lavage fluid
3. Eosinophilic infiltrate on biopsy

What is "Loffler's syndrome?"

The other name for "simple pulmonary eosinophilia"

How severe are the pulmonary symptoms in Loffler's syndrome?

They are mild

Can eosinophilic pneumonia become chronic?

Yes –
Unknown etiology

Which patient groups might develop "allergic bronchopulmonary aspergillosis?"

Those with asthma or cystic fibrosis

What occurs in allergic bronchopulmonary aspergillosis?
   (Name 3 steps)

1. Aspergillosis colonizes the bronchi

2. ↑ IgE and eosinophils

3. Worsens control of CF, asthma, and often causes bronchiectasis

"Acute" eosinophilic pneumonia is different from Loffler's syndrome. How?
   (Name 4 ways)

1. Acute febrile illness (it has acute in the name, after all)

2. *Progresses rapidly*

3. *Severe* – often leads to respiratory failure

4. Lavage has eosinophils, but blood often doesn't

What is "Churg-Strauss" syndrome?
(great distractor item!)

Asthma + vasculitis (multiorgan) + eosinophilia

What causes "Churg-Strauss?"

Unknown
(patients often have other allergic tendencies)

What is the mainstay of treatment for Churg-Strauss syndrome?

Steroids

With the exceptions of Churg-Strauss and allergic aspergillosis, what is the prognosis for the various types of eosinophilic pneumonias?

Excellent with prompt treatment when needed

What is the main complication of allergic bronchopulmonary aspergillosis (a form of eosinophilic pneumonia)?

Pulmonary fibrosis/ Severe bronchiectasis

If eosinophilic pneumonia is caused by parasites, will you be able to locate them in the stool?

Sometimes –
Several common causes are often not (e.g., toxocara, ancylostoma, early ascaris)

If the differential from the CBC does _not_ indicate eosinophilia, is eosinophilic pneumonia still a possibility?

Yes –
There may be pulmonary infiltration without peripheral eosinophilia

Steroid therapy for acute & chronic eosinophilic pneumonia is very important – What aspect requires the most careful approach?

The steroid taper must be very gradual to prevent relapse

In pediatrics, hemoptysis is most common in what age group?

Older children
&
Adolescents

What are the main things in your differential for a patient with hemoptysis?
(Name 6 general categories)

1. Bronchiectasis/pneumonia
2. Cavitary infections
3. Tumors
4. Congenital heart disease
5. Foreign body
6. Pulmonary embolus

What are the main dangers associated with significant hemoptysis?

1. Respiratory insufficiency

2. Hypovolemic shock

Why does Hanta virus cause respiratory problems?

Profound pulmonary edema

(Alveolar capillaries leak)

How do humans acquire Hantavirus?

Contact with rodent urine or feces

(wet or dry)

What are the main presenting complaints of Hantavirus infection?

High fever, headache, GI complaints

(The famous "flu-like syndrome" so many odd diseases start with)

When does cough develop for a Hantavirus patient?

When cardiac depression & pulmonary edema begin

Does a Hantavirus patient have URI complaints?

_No_!

Why are serial CBCs performed while awaiting confirmation of Hanta infection (which takes days)?

The platelet count falls in the prodromal phase – supporting the diagnosis

When pertussis infection is fatal, how does it kill?	Pneumonia *(90 % of pertussis deaths in young children are due to pneumonia)*
In general terms, why do children with pertussis develop pneumonia?	Bacterial superinfection (It is possible for pertussis to do it, directly, though)
The highest mortality for pertussis is in what age range?	<6 months (about 1 % mortality)

How is pertussis spread?
        (2 modes)
	Aerosol
	   &
	Contact with secretions

What is the common name for pertussis?	Whooping cough
Do children <6 months "whoop" with pertussis?	Usually not – Apnea is common, though (and terribly silent)
What cells does pertussis primarily attack?	Ciliated epithelium
Why does bronchiectasis develop with pertussis?	Secretions & sloughed epithelium block the bronchioles (as in RSV)
In the US, children who acquire pertussis usually encounter it in what reservoir?	Nonimmune adolescents & adults
What are the stages of B. pertussis infection?	1. Catarrhal (URI) 2. Paroxysmal (cough) 3. Convalescent (cough may continue)
What causes epiglottitis?	Various bacteria (e.g., *Hemophilus influenza* B, *Staph aureus*, *Strep pneumo*, *Strep pyogenes*)
How much has HiB vaccine decreased the incidence of epiglottitis and related HiB infections?	98 %

Strep pyogenes as a cause of epiglottitis is usually seen in what population?

School-aged children in winter/spring

Classic physical diagnostic findings for epiglottitis are?
   (Name 3)

1. Drooling
2. Tripod posture
3. "Thumb sign" on lateral neck x-ray

(The epiglottis looks like a thumb sticking into the airway)

What must never be included in the physical exam of a child suspected of having epiglottitis?

Direct visualization of the oropharynx – *Closure of the airway can result***!!!**

Should you try to send lab work on a child suspected to have epiglottitis?

Not unless the airway is secure

(Upsetting the child could cause the glottis to close)

What is the main cause of death for plague victims?

Pneumonia

How is pneumonic plague acquired?

Contact with saliva or droplet respiratory secretions (of other *humans*)

Most cases of plague occur in children & adolescents. Why?

They are more likely to have contact with rodents/small animals

Chronic, intermittent pulmonary hemorrhage can result from two autoimmune diseases. What are they?

SLE
   &
Idiopathic pulmonary hemosiderosis

Idiopathic pulmonary hemosiderosis is very similar to Goodpasture's disease. How is it different?

No effect on the kidney

Where is the hemosiderin in idiopathic pulmonary hemosiderosis?

In the macrophages (where hemosiderin is usually found!)

Do patients lose enough iron in idiopathic pulmonary hemosiderosis to become anemic?

Yes

What is the course of idiopathic pulmonary hemosiderosis?	Kids – May have spontaneous remission Adults – Chronic (Doesn't go away)
Which rheumatologic lab will be positive for Wegener's granulomatosis patients?	**c-ANCA** (p-ANCA is for polyarteritis nodosa) Mnemonic: Think of an anchor (ANCA) swinging up and sinking one end into the lungs and the other into the kidneys to remember what Wegener's affects, and that it is c-ANCA positive
What three parts of the body does Wegener's affects?	1. **Lungs** 2. **Kidneys** 3. **Upper respiratory tract/sinuses (that's why they get nosebleeds)**
What is the new term for Wegener's granulomatosis?	**Granulomatosis with polyangiitis**
What is the buzzword for the histologic changes in Wegener's granulomatosis (Granulomatosis with polyangiitis)?	**Necrotizing granulomas/ granulo-matous vasculitis**
How is a Wegener's diagnosis confirmed?	Nasal or lung biopsy (_not_ kidney biopsy – too invasive)
How do Wegener's patients usually present? (Name 3 symptoms)	• Hematuria/glomerulo-nephritis • Cough/hemoptysis • Epistaxis
Should a Wegener's patient present with dyspnea?	**No!!!**

If a patient presentation sounds like Wegener's, but Goodpasture's is also an option, how can you differentiate them? (List 4 ways – 3 are clinical 1 is lab based)	Nose stuff – Wegener's Dyspnea – Goodpasture's Anemia – Goodpasture's ANCA negative – Goodpasture's
How is Wegener's granulomatosis treated?	Cyclophosphamide ± steroids
The primary process creating the problems in Wegener's granulomatosis is _____?	Vasculitis (granulomatous type & mainly small vessel)
What is the main problem in Goodpasture's syndrome?	Antibodies to glomerular basement membrane, which deposit in both lung & kidney (*Then complement attacks it!*)
What is the buzzword for the histology in Goodpasture's?	"Linear" deposits of IgG along the basement membrane Mnemonic: Think of a one-lane road winding through a "good pasture" with a few cows & horses. This reminds you the deposits are linear in "Goodpasture's"!)
How is Goodpasture's treated?	Immunosuppressive medications & Plasmapheresis (if necessary)
How does Goodpasture's syndrome present?	Dyspnea Hemoptysis Iron deficiency anemia Glomerulonephritis
SIDS is most common in the first 6 months of life. In which of these 6 months is it very uncommon?	The first month!
Where does SIDS rank, as a cause of death in infants?	Third

What pulmonary issue is a risk factor for SIDS?

Smoking –
Both during pregnancy & passive smoke exposure after delivery

What intervention has had the biggest impact on the incidence of SIDS?

The "back to sleep" program

(Putting infants to sleep on their backs, and keeping them that way)

What two factors are most important to preventing bronchopulmonary dysplasia (BPD)?

1. **Preventing birth until** *after 30 weeks gestation*

2. **Using prenatal steroids to enhance lung development**

Which diuretic has been shown to be helpful for BPD infants?

Furosemide
(it improves lung function – others do not)

After birth, are steroids helpful in the management of BPD?

<u>No</u>

What is the mainstay of treatment for BPD, and how do you know whether it is effective?

• **Oxygen (low flow)**
• **Weight gain (20–40 g per day)**

Infants with pulmonary conditions like BPD are sometimes given RSV immunoglobulin. If RSV-IVIG is given, how does this alter the infant's immunization schedule?

MMR & Varicella vaccines cannot be given until *9 months after the last IVIG*

What is the difference in onset for broncho-pulmonary dysplasia vs. bronchiolitis obliterans?

• BPD must begin within roughly 1 month of birth

• Bronchiolitis obliterans usually occurs between 6 months and 2 years, and *follows an infection*

What *is* bronchiolitis obliterans?

Small airways close up → poor gas exchange

Which ethnic group is at special risk to develop bronchiolitis obliterans?

Native Americans

Which infection is especially likely to *produce* bronchiolitis obliterans?

Adenovirus lower respiratory infection

(Especially types 3, 7 & 21 Mnemonic: 3 × 7 = 21)

In addition to gas exchange problems, producing hypoxemia & hypercarbia, what other respiratory problem often develops for bronchiolitis obliterans patients?

Pulmonary edema

How is bronchiolitis obliterans diagnosed definitively?

Lung biopsy

If a child has adenovirus pneumonia, what is the probability that he or she will develop bronchiolitis obliterans?

1/3!!!

(For Native Americans, about 2/3)

In addition to adenovirus infection, what other situations increase the risk of bronchiolitis obliterans?

Lung transplant
   Or
Bone marrow transplantation with Graft vs. Host Disease (GVHD)

Is bronchiolitis obliterans related to BOOP (bronchiolitis obliterans organizing pneumonia)?

No

Which patient age group is at highest risk to develop BOOP?

Adults –
Although it does occur in kids

How is the pathology different in the two bronchiolitis obliterans disorders?

BO – Loss of patency in the smallest airways leads to reduced surfaces for gas exchange

BOOP – Hyperplasia & inflammatory infiltrates swell the respiratory septa, blocking the small airways

How do BOOP patients present clinically?

Multiple bouts of bronchitis that <u>do</u> respond to antibiotics

Which cells are hyperplastic in BOOP?

Type II pneumocytes

(The ones that make surfactant, remember?)

What is the best known disorder involving respiratory cilia dysfunction?	**Kartagener's**
What is the nature of the problem with the cilia in Kartagener's disorder?	**One or both of the "dynein arms" that make the cilium move are missing**
Is Kartagener's syndrome common or rare?	**Rare**
What are the presentations of Kartagener's syndrome? (Name 4)	Sinusitis Bronchiectasis Male infertility Situs inversus (!)
Are antibiotics indicated in most cases of foreign body aspiration?	**No – Just get it out!**
What is the probability that an aspirated foreign body won't be diagnosed for a month after the incident (in pediatrics)?	**1 in 5 (Yikes!)**
Which objects are the most popular ones for aspiration, among children?	**Seeds & nuts (including peanuts)**
If most aspirated foreign bodies are radiolucent, why is a chest x-ray helpful for diagnosis?	**Most (about 2/3) will have localized hyperinflation noticeable on x-ray**
If a child has aspirated an object, and you're not sure what it is, should you try a blind finger sweep?	No! (You might push the object further in.)
What is bronchiectasis, when it occurs as a chronic condition?	Dilatation or distortion of the bronchi
How do patients with chronic bronchiectasis present?	• Recurrent pulmonary infections • Chronic productive cough • Wheezing • Clubbing (very common)

How would a child develop bronchiectasis?	Infection or inflammation
Define "periodic breathing?" (Name 3 components)	Pause of ≥ 3 s At least three times Less than 20 s of respiration between each episode
No breathing for how many seconds <u>definitely</u> constitutes apnea?	20 s
When does failure to breathe for less than 20 s *still* constitute apnea?	If cyanosis or bradycardia occurs along with the pause
Periodic breathing is most normal & common in which infant group?	Preemies
Is prematurity a risk factor for SIDS?	Yes
Is apnea of prematurity a risk factor for SIDS?	No!!!
If an asthma patient has an abnormal sinus x-ray, is it safe to assume that antibiotic therapy is indicated?	No – Most kids with asthma have abnormal sinus x-rays
Which asthma medication decreases lower esophageal sphincter tone, possibly worsening GE reflux and increasing the possibility of asthma exacerbations?	Theophylline
What treatment is most recommended for children with exercise-induced asthma?	Short acting β-adrenergic med just before exercise
If asthma symptoms are well controlled on the current regimen, when should the patient have follow-up, and what is the goal of follow-up?	• Follow-up in 1–6 months after good control is established • Evaluate for possible "step-down" in treatment

What is the most critical, simple, measure for the long-term management of asthma?	**A peak flow meter (& proper knowledge of how to use it)**
Do inhaled steroids have the same long-term side effects as the systemic steroids?	**Generally, no**
What class of agents are salmeterol and formoterol?	Long-acting β_2-agonists (12 h action)
What is the very important limitation to the use of salmeterol and formoterol?	*Not* useful in acute asthma (long acting <u>and slow onset</u>)
Which common CNS drugs will decrease theophylline levels?	**Phenobarbital & Phenytoin**
Ciprofloxacin elevates theophylline levels. Which two common pediatric medications will also elevate theophylline levels?	**Erythromycin & Cimetidine**
Recurrent or prolonged croup could be a manifestation of what congenital tracheal malformation?	**Tracheal stenosis (usually segmental)**
If an infant has significant tracheal stenosis at birth, how will he or she present?	**Severe retractions, stridor & dyspnea**
Webs can sometimes partly or completely obstruct the laryngeal inlet. What genetic syndrome are they associated with?	**Velocardiofacial syndrome**
What genetic problem should you test for in an infant with glottic webs?	**22q11**
What are laryngeal cysts?	Pouches of mucus-secreting epithelium, usually supraglottic

What causes laryngeal cysts?	Usually result from trauma or prolonged intubation (removed via laser)
How does subglottic stenosis present?	**Congenital – stridor in first few months** **Acquired – follows multiple intubations/procedures, often asymptomatic**
How can you evaluate whether your patient has subglottic stenosis?	Bronchoscopy is best, but direct laryngoscopy can provide diagnosis & some limited information
How is congenital subglottic stenosis managed?	Nothing if asymptomatic Surgery as early as possible if symptomatic
What is the most common cause of stridor in the newborn?	**Laryngomalacia**
At what age is laryngomalacia most often symptomatic?	2 weeks
How is laryngomalacia managed?	Most kids outgrow it by about 1 year
What is congenital lobar emphysema, and which part of the lung is most often affected?	• One or more lobes abnormally enlarged & filled with *air or fluid* • Left upper lobe
When do infants with congenital lobar emphysema present?	Birth to 6 months old
Which infants are most likely to have pulmonary hypoplasia, in terms of their birth history?	**Premature due to premature rupture of membranes**
How is pulmonary hypoplasia managed?	**Support oxygenation via mechanical ventilation or ECMO until lungs grow**
Is pulmonary hypoplasia a common reason for neonatal infant death?	**Yes**

What is a pulmonary sequestration?	**An area of nonfunctional lung-type tissue either within the lung or outside it. It has its own arterial supply & venous drainage.**
Will a bronchoscopy help you to diagnose a sequestration?	**No –** **It is not part of the normal airway architecture, so you won't see it**
What will help you to diagnose a pulmonary sequestration, in terms of radiology evaluations?	**CT scan or Chest x-ray** **(Doppler US can sometimes be used due to the abnormal vessels serving the sequestration)**
What is scimitar syndrome? *(Great distracter item!)*	**When right pulmonary venous blood returns to the IVC**
There are two forms of scimitar syndrome, labeled infantile & adult. What is the difference?	Adult: Appears later (childhood or adolescence) Has a better prognosis Involves just a small amount of right pulmonary blood returning to the IVC
How does the infantile form of scimitar syndrome present?	Respiratory distress & Heart failure (Bad prognosis)
How would a pulmonary sequestration patient present?	1. **Respiratory distress** 2. **Bad pleuritic chest pain** 3. **Hemoptysis** 4. **Recurrent pneumonia**
Patients with pulmonary A-V fistulas most likely have what autosomal dominant disorder?	**Osler-Weber-Rendu** (aka hereditary hemorrhagic telangiectasia) Mnemonic: Think of a gentleman all dressed up dancing the "rendu," an old-fashioned dance. Unfortunately he gets a nosebleed and also bright red blood per rectum, because these patients have lots of hemorrhagic telangiectasias

A child with asthma & nasal polyps is likely to have a medication sensitivity to what drug?	**Aspirin** (It's called the "aspirin triad" & sometimes also called "Samter's triad")
If a bronchogenic cyst is identified, is it okay to observe it as long as it is asymptomatic?	No – Excision is better due to the potential for malignancy & likely symptoms from local compression (eventually) or infection
Why do bronchogenic cysts increase in size over time?	They are usually mucous filled & more is secreted over time
In addition to compressing nearby structures, why else do bronchogenic cysts become symptomatic?	Infection → Chest pain, fever, & cough
At what amount of curvature do you expect scoliosis to affect pulmonary function?	**50°** **(the problem is usually alveolar hypoventilation)**
What causes scoliosis, in most cases?	**Idiopathic** **(we don't know)** *Early bracing will fix it*
Cardiopulmonary compromise is expected when scoliosis reaches what level?	90°
Does pectus excavatum cause pulmonary problems? (Pectus excavatum means the chest goes inward)	**No** (Repair is cosmetic only)
Pectus carinatum is when the sternum is unusually far out, and the lateral parts of the rib cage are flattened (pigeon chest). Does it cause pulmonary problems?	**No** (Repair is cosmetic only)
Jeune syndrome alters the rib cage so that it is smaller than usual. Does this cause pulmonary problems?	Yes – Restrictive lung disease & frequent infections

Jeune syndrome always causes short ribs, small rib cage, and what other problem?

Renal disease

Jeune syndrome patients often have a variety of musculoskeletal issues and are always affected by a small rib cage & renal disease. How does Jeune syndrome develop?

Autosomal recessive disorder

Mnemonic:
"Recessive-renal-rib cage" on a *young* dwarf. (Jeune means young in French, and Jeune syndrome patients sometimes also have dwarfism. Visualize a kidney inside a "receding" rib cage on the poor young dwarf.)

What is the other name for jeune syndrome (the descriptive name)?

Asphyxiating
Thoracic
Dystrophy

What is the most common lethal recessive disorder?

Cystic Fibrosis

What is the second most common lethal recessive disorder?

**SMA
(Spinal Muscular Atrophy)**

Why do the spinal muscles atrophy in SMA?

Degeneration of the anterior horn nuclei (sometimes also the bulbar nuclei)

Where is the gene for spinal muscular atrophy?

Chromosome 5q

Will patients with SMA develop sensory or cognitive problems?

**No –
The anterior horn cells (& sometimes bulbar nuclei) are the only ones affected, so it is *motor only***

Which famous infectious disease also kills off the anterior horn cells of the spinal cord?

Polio

(So SMA patients look much like polio patients!)

If SMA is such a common and deadly disease, why haven't I heard more about it?

There are three forms –
The worst (& best known) one is Werdnig-Hoffman –
You've probably heard of that

How can you remember which gene causes the SMA group of disorders?	• **Because they symmetrically weaken the muscles of "all 5" extremities – arms, legs, & head (if the bulbar nuclei are affected)**
	• **& it makes the patient "queer" ("q" part of the chromosome) in their motor function, not petite (p)!**
What are the three types of SMA?	• Werdnig-Hoffman is Type I (aka Severe Infantile)
	• Intermediate or Chronic Infantile is Type II
	• Mild SMA is Type III (aka Kugelberg-Welander)
	(The main info to know is that there are three types, and that Werdnig-Hoffman is Type I)
Is CPK normal or elevated with SMA?	**Normal –** **Muscle degeneration is secondary to nerve degeneration**
	(CPK goes up when muscle damage is the primary problem)
Are proximal or distal muscles more affected in Werdnig-Hoffman, and the other types of SMA?	**Proximal** **(& legs are more affected than arms)**
How does Werdnig-Hoffman present?	• **<6 months old** • **Hypotonia/weakness** • **Difficulty feeding** • *Tongue fasciculations*!
How easy is it to diagnose SMA disorders with genetic screening for chromosome 5q mutations?	**Pretty easy –** **95 % will be found**
Biochemically, what causes Duchenne muscular dystrophy?	**Missing or deficient dystrophin (a muscle protein)**
How is Duchenne muscular dystrophy inherited?	**X-linked** (recessive)

What finding usually precedes significant motor function problems in Duchenne's?

Scoliosis

(worsens rapidly after the child is wheelchair bound)

At what age will boys with muscular dystrophy begin to have problems? What are the usual problems?
  (Name 3 examples)

Ages 2–6 years

(Think "frequent falling," "toe-walking," and "waddling gait")

Is CPK elevated in Duchenne's?

(very frequent item)

Yes –
The muscle cells are having problems, so CPK is high

What two buzzwords on physical exam & history go with Duchenne's?

(very frequent item)

1. **Calf pseudo-hypertrophy (they look big)**

2. **Gower's sign – using the hands to rise or "pushing up" the legs with the arms to stand**

How is the diagnosis of Duchenne's made?

Muscle biopsy

Is the muscle dysfunction of Duchenne's limited to the lower extremities?

No –
All skeletal muscle is affected, & *cardiomyopathy is also a big problem*

Long-term, what type of problem usually ends the lives of Duchenne's patients?

Respiratory –
Respiratory muscle weakness → respiratory failure + aspiration/ pulmonary infection is common due to weak bulbar muscles

Is there any effective therapy for Duchenne's?

No –
Supportive only

Neonatal myasthenia gravis can compromise the infant's respira- tions. What *is* **neonatal myasthenia?**

Antibodies from the mom's myasthenia are circulating in the baby → muscle weakness

How do neonatal myasthenia patients present?

Same as usual –
Ptosis, hypotonia, weak cry, difficulty feeding

What is the course of neonatal myasthenia gravis?	It resolves during or after the neonatal period (as the antibodies are destroyed)
Is congenital myasthenia the same as neonatal myasthenia?	No! (*Can you believe that?!*)
How can you recognize congenital myasthenia gravis?	No antibodies (to the acetylcholine receptor)
What is congenital myasthenia, then?	An autosomal recessive disorder with *variable* age of onset – Abnormal acetylcholine receptors cause a myasthenia-like syndrome
"Regular" myasthenia, when it occurs in the pediatric population is called _____?	Juvenile myasthenia gravis
What diagnostic test can be used to confirm the diagnosis when myasthenia is suspected?	Edrophonium/the Tensilon Test (It is an anticholinesterase medication, so it boosts acetylcholine levels – function should improve briefly.)
What is the problem in myasthenia gravis (neonatal, juvenile, or adult forms)?	Antibodies to the acetylcholine receptor decrease muscle strength/ function
Increasing use of muscles in myasthenic patients produces what result?	*Increasing* weakness
How is myasthenia gravis treated medically?	Anticholinesterase medications (oral) & Immunosuppression
What surgical management technique produces remission in about 50 % of myasthenia patients?	Thymectomy
Is juvenile-onset myasthenia gravis more common in girls or boys?	Girls (like most autoimmune disorders)
What is eventration?	Significant elevation of a hemidiaphragm

What is the typical cause of eventration?

Usually congenital

(can be acquired via phrenic nerve injury)

Is eventration more common in boys or girls?

Boys

(Usually on the left side)

Accessory diaphragm (an extra diaphragm-like tissue in one hemithorax) usually causes what symptoms or signs?

- Respiratory distress due to lung hypoplasia in neonates
- Recurrent infections in older kids

If a disorder has "dystrophy" in the name, what does that mean about the disorder (e.g., muscular dystrophy)?

There is defective production of an important molecule – due to a nutrition or metabolism problem

Pneumonia almost never occurs without what sign?

Fever

When is it reasonable to get blood cultures in a child suspected or known to have pneumonia?

For patients requiring admission with very significant cases of pneumonia

(Note: The federal government is now forcing us to send cultures for pneumonia patients – this is not medically indicated, however.)

If you suspect a patient has pneumonia, is it a good idea to send an ESR and/or CRP?

No – not helpful

Should serological tests, as well as cold agglutinins and viral studies, be ordered when pneumonia is suspected?

**Generally no –
Not unless it would change management**

If you're not sure whether a pneumonia merits antibiotic therapy, what test(s) might help you decide?

**CBC –
Check for WBCs >15,000
(more likely to be bacterial)**

If you're not sure whether the patient has a pneumonia, what test may help you decide?

CXR, of course

(Does not tell you whether it's bacterial or viral, though)

When is it reasonable to order a chest x-ray in cases of suspected childhood pneumonia?
(3)

1. **Pneumonia unresponsive to antibiotics**
2. **Pleural effusion is suspected**
3. **High fever & ↑ WBCs without a source in a child <5 years old**

In addition to fever, what other sign is a very important predictor of a (severe) pneumonia?

Cyanosis

Signs of respiratory distress are most likely to indicate that a child has pneumonia when the child has more than one of them. What group of signs should you be looking for?
(5)

Cough
Tachypnea
Crackles
Decreased breath sounds
Retractions

Pneumonia is hardest to diagnose in which age group?

<2 years old

What is the usual course for pleural effusions that develop in response to an infection?

Spontaneous resolution (although it may take weeks)

Recurrence of fever or respiratory symptoms in a child with a recently resolved pneumonia should make you consider what diagnosis?

Empyema

(An infected pleural effusion)

How is an empyema treated?

Drain the fluid and give antibiotics

Early in the course of streptococcal pneumonia, what are you supposed to hear on auscultatory exam?

Pleural friction rub
(crackles come later)

How are empyemas usually drained?

Initial thoracentesis, then closed suction drainage

Strep pyogenes is Group A Strep. When it causes pneumonia, what will the patient's history usually be?

A rash disease (e.g., rubeola, scarlet fever, or varicella), then pneumonia developed

Which lung abnormality often develops with Strep pyogenes pneumonia?

Pneumatocele

(resolves spontaneously)

Which two types of pneumonia often produce pneumatoceles?	*Strep pyogenes* & *Staph aureus*
Klebsiella is most likely to affect which pediatric patient populations? (2)	Prolonged intubation & Immunocompromised
***Staph aureus* pneumonia usually develops with what history?**	**Recent viral URI or influenza**
Which patients are at greatest risk for anaerobic pneumonias?	Patients who aspirate (rare otherwise)
What is the usual drug of choice for anaerobic pneumonias?	**Clindamycin**
Histoplasmosis is common in which parts of the US?	**Mississippi & Ohio River Valleys** (In other words, midwestern and mid-southern US)
Histoplasmosis is associated with which creatures?	Bats & Birds (& soil with bat or bird droppings)
What is the usual course for histoplasmosis infection?	**Most are asymptomatic**
Bad cases of histoplasmosis require what treatment?	**Amphotericin B** **(It's a fungus! Bad fungus gets Ampho B)**
A patient presents with erythema multiforme, history of travel to the southwest US, and chest x-ray shows "thin-walled" blebs. What's the diagnosis?	**Coccidioidomycosis**
Coccidioidomycosis + worsening chest x-ray or hemoptysis =	**Treatment –** **Use Ampho B or Fluconazole** (*most cases don't require treatment, though*)

When coccidioidomycosis occurs in immuno-compromised or HIV patients, how does it often manifest?

Fulminant & often fatal –
Bone, skin, & meningeal involvement

Multiple "masses" on chest x-ray, and large yeast with single buds on sputum sample, mean your patient has what infectious disease?

Blastomycosis

Mnemonic:
Single Bud Blasto –
Just use the sounds or imagine a single guy named "Bud" who has no success with the ladies. They always tell him to "blast-off!"

In children, blastomycosis sometimes disseminates to what two areas (from the lungs)?

Bone
&
Skin

Mnemonic:
Blasto goes to Bone &
KidS SKin

Where is blastomycosis usually found in the United States?

**Midwest
&
Midatlantic/Southeastern**

(Think of a stripe from Connecticut southward, and Chicago southward)

If a blastomycosis pneumonia patient is having a mild course, what should you do in terms of treatment?

Observe

(also okay to give oral itraconazole)

Which fungal pneumonia is also known as San Joaquin Valley Fever?

Coccidioidomycosis

Mnemonic:
The San Joaquin Valley is in California. "C" is for Coccidioides!

How is allergic bronchopulmonary aspergillosis treated?

Corticosteroids

What unusual chest x-ray appearance is sometimes noted with allergic bronchopulmonary aspergillosis?

Not only do infiltrates migrate, sometimes there is also an *infiltrate that looks like "fingers in a glove" in the central lung (creepy!)*

Do atypical pneumonia patients usually have a productive cough?	No
If a patient develops an atypical pneumonia – and the vignette mentions that the patient participated in hunting or skinning animals – which atypical pneumonia does he or she have?	Tularemia
Your patient has an *atypical pneumonia*, and the vignette mentions that they've been around *cattle or sheep*. What's the diagnosis?	Q fever (caused by *Coxiella burnetii*)
Is *Coxiella burnetii* pulmonary infection contagious between people?	No
What is the most common cause of community acquired pneumonia for kids >5 years old?	Mycoplasma
Is atypical pneumonia common in pre-school children?	No – Generally seen ages 6 years & up
Is a positive cold agglutinin test diagnostic for mycoplasma?	Not diagnostic – It is suggestive, though
What lab test is definitive for mycoplasma infection, when positive?	IgM serology
What problems outside the lung sometimes develop in ENT systems with mycoplasma infection?	Pharyngitis Tonsillitis *Bullous myringitis* (vesicles on the tympanic membrane)
Mycoplasma infection sometimes causes neurological problems. What neurological sign is especially associated with mycoplasma infection?	Confusion

What rheumatological issues can mycoplasma infection induce?	**Arthritis (of course)** & **Erythema multiforme** (& occasionally the more serious Stevens-Johnson syndrome with lesions on mucous membranes)
What effects does Mycoplasma sometimes have on the hematological system?	**Hemolytic anemia** & **Splenomegaly**
If you can't use a macrolide to treat mycoplasma (due to allergy, etc.), what inexpensive alternative could you use?	**Doxycycline!** (Fine for Chlamydia & many other atypicals, too – avoid in children <7 years due to tooth issues)
Chlamydia pneumonia has another name – **what is it?**	**TWAR pneumonia** **Or** **TWAR pathogen** (TW & AR designate the labs that originally found the organism. That's how it got the name "TWAR")
Is an epidemic of atypical pneumonia likely to be caused by Chlamydia or Mycoplasma?	**Chlamydia**
What unusual pattern does chlamydial pneumonia often follow?	Sore throat that resolves, then, Pneumonia 2–3 weeks later
How rapidly does Mycoplasma infection spread?	Slowly (2–3-week incubation period)
What is the preferred regimen for mild persistent asthma? **(Episodes >2× per week, but not every day)**	**Inhaled corticosteroid** **(daily)**
In moderate persistent asthma, how frequent are the asthma problems?	**Daily** (*That's why they call it persistent, it happens every day*)

What is the preferred treatment regimen for patients with moderate persistent asthma?
(Name 2 options)

Medium-dose inhaled steroids
   Or
Low-dose inhaled steroids &
long-acting inhaled β-agonist

If your patient has moderate persistent asthma, but the episodes are worse than average, or the patient develops severe exacerbations regularly, what slightly stronger than usual regimen may be required?

Medium-dose inhaled steroids
   &
Long-acting inhaled β-agonist

How would you identify a patient with severe persistent asthma?

Continuous day-time difficulties with asthma

(& frequent problems at night)

What is the recommended treatment for severe persistent asthma?
(minimum required)

High-dose inhaled steroids
   &
Long-acting inhaled β-agonist

In addition to the inhaled medication regimen for severe persistent asthma, some patients may also need what treatment?

Oral steroids

(2 mg/kg/day up to 60 mg)

Which asthma patients are candidates for leukotriene inhibitors?

Mild & moderate asthma patients

If you choose to use a leukotriene inhibitor for your patient with moderate asthma, what other medication must be part of the regimen?

Inhaled corticosteroids

(*A leukotriene can be used by itself can be used in mild persistent disease*)

Which type of asthma has an "intermittent" form?

Only mild!!!

(otherwise, it's all some sort of persistent asthma)

Stridor that is both inspiratory & expiratory usually indicates that the patient has what disorder?

Subglottic stenosis

(congenital or acquired)

If a patient has both inspiratory & expiratory stridor, which component is usually louder?	Inspiratory
What causes expiratory stridor?	Problems below the thoracic inlet (trachea or bronchi)
If something is compressing the trachea, expiratory stridor often results. What other pulmonary exam finding is common?	Wheezing
Tracheomalacia means "soft trachea." What is the practical consequence of tracheomalacia during breathing?	The trachea collapses during expiration
Stridor just during inspiration, with a quiet expiration in an otherwise well infant, is most often due to _____?	**Laryngomalacia**
If a child is presented who has expiratory stridor _and feeding problems_, what diagnosis should leap to mind?	**Extrinsic tracheal & esophageal compression _due to vascular ring_** (It encircles both)
If you suspect that your expiratory stridor patient with feeding difficulties has a vascular ring problem, how can you evaluate that possibility?	Barium swallow study
A child is presented with expiratory stridor, and the vignette mentions that a tracheo-esophageal fistula repair was done in infancy. What is the likely cause of the expiratory stridor?	**Tracheomalacia – It is a common long-term complication of TE fistula repair**
When might a tracheomalacia patient present with "biphasic" stridor? (Biphasic means both inspiratory & expiratory)	**If the problem is very high (near the larynx)**

Can pulsus paradoxus be a sign of respiratory failure?	**Yes** **(Inspiration vs. expiration SBP difference >10 mmHg)**
If a vignette asks you to make a decision about whether intubation is needed, what is the "first thing" you need to do?	**Assess respiratory effort/assess the airway**
Is a normal respiratory rate reassuring when evaluating for possible respiratory failure?	**Not by itself –** **Can mean that a tachypneic patient has fatigued to a normal rate**
If you are evaluating for possible impending respiratory failure, how reliable are sweating & tachycardia?	**Not great, because they are also signs of anxiety**
What is the earliest sign of impending respiratory failure?	**Tachypnea**

In addition to tachypnea, when it is present, what are other good signs of impending respiratory failure?
    (Name 2 signs)
	Retractions
	    &
	Pulsus paradoxus
	(SBP drop >10 mmHg with inspiration)

Headache, joint pain, unexpected clot formation & hemoptysis should make you think of what pulmonary-related disorder?	Polycythemia due to chronic hypoxemia
In addition to the increase in hematocrit, what other change in the CBC accompanies polycythemia?	Platelets are destroyed more rapidly – ↑ bleeding risk & low platelets
Are cough suppressants a good idea?	No – None have been shown to be better than placebo
Which patients often do not cough well enough to clear their respiratory passages? (Name 3 categories)	1. Nerve & muscle disorder patients (vocal cord paralysis, CP, etc.) 2. Those in pain 3. Thoracic deformities

On the boards, a parent asks whether it would be alright to give a 6-year-old a cough suppressant to help him sleep. What is the correct response?

No –
Not effective as it s a newly popular to test item "& risks medication side effects!"

Appropriate tests at the initial evaluation of a kid with a chronic cough are _____?
   (Name 3 tests)

1. TB test
2. Chest x-ray
3. Sweat test

A cough that disappears during sleep is usually due to what?

Psychogenic

(often loud & brassy cough when kid is awake)

What is the "buzz phrase" that often goes with psychogenic cough?

Can be "produced on command"

What is the current trend for mortality from asthma?

Increasing

If a child has mild asthma, what is the likelihood that he or she will outgrow it with age?

60 %

For children with severe asthma, what is the likelihood of outgrowing the asthma?

30 %

(Still pretty good, considering…)

Which is more effective – MDI with spacer or nebulizer?

Equal in children old enough to use them properly

(MDI = metered-dose inhaler)

Which gender has more asthma?

Boys before puberty –
Girls after

In an asthma patient having an asthma episode, is a normal CO_2 a good thing?

No –
Should be low due to rapid breathing

Chronic nighttime cough without associated symptoms or history is likely to be what disorder?

Asthma

If a nighttime cough is productive, but without other symptoms or history, is asthma still likely?	**Yes**
In addition to asthma, what other causes of nighttime cough should you consider? **(Name 2 causes)**	**GE reflux** **Sinusitis**
Infants that wheeze may have asthma (assuming it's not due to an infection), but what other important structural & environmental problems should you consider? **(Name 3 problems)**	**Aspiration of something** **Vascular ring** **BPD (Bronchopulmonary dysplasia)**
If a child has allergies, how much more likely is he/she to develop asthma than kids without allergies?	3×
If a vignette tells you that a child is "having trouble exercising," what differential should you run through?	<u>C</u>ardiac problems <u>A</u>nemia <u>M</u>uscle disorder <u>P</u>sychology/<u>P</u>ulmonary factors (e.g., depression) **Mnemonic:** **Think of a kid having trouble exercising at CAMPP!**
What is the main concern with giving steroids to children long-term?	Growth problems (other concerns: hypertension, osteoporosis, & cataracts)
Why are inhaled steroids the preferred method for preventing asthma exacerbations, in terms of their actions on the pulmonary system?	Decreases inflammation & Bronchial hyperreactivity
What about the onset of reactive airway disease can help you to predict whether it will continue or spontaneously resolve?	Very early onset (<3 years) is *more likely to resolve*

A family history of asthma in which parent makes persistent asthma more likely?

Mother

What lab abnormalities suggest that your patient will probably keep asthma into adulthood?

↑ IgE
   &
Eosinophilia

On a CF sweat test, what number is a positive test?

60 mEq

(*Sometimes normal values are included in boards vignettes, so you need to know!*)

What lab abnormalities should make you suspicious that a child might have CF?
   (two main ones)

Low albumin
Low sodium

Can CF carriers sometimes have mild manifestations of CF, due to their carrier state?

No!

Don't be fooled by this one! Popular item

Has DNA testing replaced sweat testing as the gold standard for CF diagnosis?

No

In infancy, which symptoms of CF are more prominent – gut or lung symptoms?

Gut

If your patient has CF, what are the chances that his/her healthy sibling is a carrier?

2/3

(Remember it's a *healthy* sibling, so she/he can only be a carrier or have two completely normal genes. That's why it's 2 out of 3.)

What is the CF carrier rate in the general Caucasian US population?

1 in 25

If the healthy sibling of a CF patient marries someone from the general population, what is the probability that their first child will have CF?	1 in 150 (Easier to memorize than to calculate, for most of us. 2/3 probability carrier x 1/25 probability carrier in population x 1/4 probability child gets both bad genes)
Which vitamin supplement is especially important for children with CF?	Vitamin E
Are infections in CF patients eliminated with antibiotic treatment, or just controlled?	Controlled
What neuro problems sometimes develop in CF patients as a consequence of gut problems/vitamin malabsorption?	Ptosis Truncal ataxia Problems with proprioception
Vitamin absorption issues can lead to what hematologic problem for CF patients?	Bleeding – Vitamin K deficiency
If cor pulmonale develops due to partial airway obstruction, will it reverse if you fix the airway problem?	Yes
If cor pulmonale develops due to pulmonary hypertension, can it be reversed?	Generally not
Lower extremity edema, hepatomegaly, gallop heart rhythm, and sometimes clubbing, suggest what diagnosis?	Cor pulmonale
Hypoproteinemia, anemia, and steatorrhea in an infant often indicates what diagnosis?	**CF**
If a pneumonia patient improves with treatment initially, then stays sick or worsens, suspect what diagnosis?	**Empyema**

A vignette patient is described as "*cyanotic* with a *depressed sensorium*." What conclusion are you expected to draw that explains both findings?
(Don't think too deeply!)

Patient is hypoxic

If a vignette patient has "*headaches*," and is described as "*flushed and agitated*," the boards may be trying to indicate that the patient has what pulmonary-related problem?

Hypercapnia

(elevated CO_2 will vasodilate intracerebral vessels → headache)

Does sarcoidosis always create respiratory symptoms?

No

Weight loss, fatigue, and hilar adenopathy is probably a description of which disorder?

Sarcoid

Sarcoid & tuberculosis have some similarities. Both can affect the heart. How does each affect the heart?

TB – pericarditis

Sarcoid – conduction changes (blocks or widening of components)

A child who refuses to lie down, prefers to sit leaning forward, has dysphonia, dysphagia, drooling, & stridor has what diagnosis?

Epiglottitis

(*more likely is child is not H. flu immunized*)

Do epiglottitis patients have a cough?

No

What kind of stridor do epiglottitis patients tend to have, if they have stridor?

Biphasic

(the swelling is just supraglottic, so it can cause noise in both directions)

If you suspect epiglottitis, and you'd like to get pre-op labs, should you order them (after all, the patient is going to the OR for intubation)?

No –
Let them draw labs after intubation – the airway sometimes closes off when the child cries

Chylothorax (lymphatic fluid leaking into the thorax) most often happens in what setting?

Post-surgical

(especially following cardiovascular and scoliosis surgery)

Which two values are high in the lab analysis of chylous fluid?

Triglycerides (>110)
Protein (>3)

If a pleural effusion is a "transudate," what does that mean, in general terms?

The fluid developed due to a problem that was not directly a lung problem

What are some typical causes of a transudate?
   (Name 3 causes)

1. CHF
2. Nephrotic syndrome
3. Cirrhosis

How high do you expect triglycerides to be if the fluid is a transudate?

Low (<50)

If an adolescent develops a spontaneous pneumothorax, what predisposing factors should you be thinking about?

1. **Connective tissue disorders (although tall think male adolescents have a higher chance of spontaneous pneumothorax even if they are perfectly healthy)**

2. **Marijuana use – The huge inhalation, and attempting to hold the smoke in, can lead to pneumothorax**

Is there a correlation between the amount of pain a patient feels and the severity of a pneumothorax?

No

In some cases, a small but significant pneumothorax can be treated with what minimally invasive treatment?

Needle aspiration

(*pneumothorax of about 15 %*)

What are the three most common causes of croup?

1. Parainfluenza
2. Influenza
3. RSV

If an infant has an ALTE (apparent life-threatening event), what is the correct disposition for the patient?

Admit for observation & evaluation

(*The infant is fine at the time of exam.*)

An ALTE always involves what
history?

1. Stopped breathing
2. Turned pale or blue & unresponsive
3. Got better (resuscitates with
   stimulation, mouth-to-mouth, etc.)

What are the main causes to evaluate
in an ALTE patient?

Trauma/abuse
Pulmonary
Neuro

Reflux/aspiration
Electrolyte
Infection

Mnemonic:
Think of an infant on a camping trip in
the wilderness with a problem. If the
infant has an apparent life-threatening
event, she/he could need a lot of support
– like TPN from REI, the wilderness
outfitters!

Is pulse oximetry a reliable measure
of oxygenation for a patient in shock?

Not really –
Peripheral vasculature is "clamped
down" so blood flow is limited

If a patient's blood is described as
being "chocolate colored," what
diagnosis should you suspect?

Methemoglobinemia

If a patient's blood is described as
being "cherry red," what diagnosis
should you suspect?

Carbon monoxide poisoning

Can the pulse oximeter produce a
reliable estimate of oxygenation with
carboxyhemoglobin circulating?

No

(It will just read that the hemoglobin is
bound, but not whether it is bound to
oxygen vs. carbon monoxide.)

Will anemic patients have reliable
pulse ox measurements?

Not if the hemoglobin is very low (<6)

RSV is the most common cause of
bronchiolitis. What is the second most
common cause?

Parainfluenza

What is the best way to prevent RSV transmission to other patients?
A – put a mask on the infected patient
B – put a mask on the other patients
C – wash hands frequently

C – Wash hands
(the board exam likes hand washing)

A *mentally retarded child* presents with *sudden onset* of a *nonproductive cough*. The child has a history of asthma, and is *wheezing* on the *right side only*. Likely diagnosis?

Foreign body aspiration

(The exam often throws in some red herring pulmonary stuff like this.)

In what proportion of foreign body aspirations do the parents or child report an aspiration event?

½

Recurrent lower respiratory tract infections with atelectasis developing in the same area each time suggests what diagnosis?

Bronchiectasis

What clue to the bronchiectasis diagnosis can you often find in the history of the cough?

Cough symptoms vary with position

What is the best way to make the bronchiectasis diagnosis?

Chest CT

Most children who catch TB are asymptomatic. How helpful is a chest x-ray for diagnosing TB in kids?

When it's positive, it's helpful, *but it's often negative in children*

(The CXR is often as asymptomatic as the child)

A child is brought in for low-grade fever & cough for 6 weeks. On exam, the child seems well, but has rales at the bases. What is the likely diagnosis?

TB – Active

(Start triple therapy until sensitivities are available)

If you are treating TB meningitis, should you use steroids?

Yes

If a patient is diagnosed with TB meningitis, what treatment should you start?

Triples (Rifampin, INH, & Pyrazinamide)
    +
Streptomycin

Streptomycin is discontinued when INH sensitivity is confirmed

What is disseminated TB called (when it spreads all over, and especially to the lungs, as many tiny foci of TB)?

Miliary TB

Mnemonic:
"Miliary" refers to millet seeds – so think of TB sprinkled like seeds throughout the body

If a child has symptoms of what seems to be a bacterial pneumonia, but also has an effusion & is an immigrant, what will you need to consider?

Pleural effusion can be primary TB

If a child has had chest trauma, and is tachycardic with signs of respiratory distress, what is the most important procedure to perform?

Physical exam comes first
(at least a brief exam)

If the answer choices for a board exam question have "perform physical exam" as an option, why is that important?

It is very often the right answer!

What is the initial chest x-ray appearance of ARDS?

"Fine, diffuse, reticular infiltrate"

What is the main problem in ARDS?

Wet alveoli –
The alveolar capillaries are too leaky → pulmonary edema

What two ventilator parameters are important for improving the respiratory status of your ARDS patient?

• PEEP
• Low tidal volume

Assuming the pulmonary situation can be handled in ARDS, why is the mortality for these patients still relatively high?

Often develops into multi-system organ failure
(liver, kidneys, etc., deteriorate)

If a male patient is noted to have atresia or absence of the vas deferens, what is the most likely underlying cause?

CF

What nasal test is sometimes used to aid in the diagnosis of CF?

Nasal potential difference measurement (as in electrical potential – it is altered due to the unusual sodium concentration in CF)

What happens chemically to make the secretions of CF patients so thick?
  (Name 2)

• **Overactive sodium pumps**

• **Chloride channels that are blocked in epithelial tissue**

Which factor correlates most strongly to lifespan in CF patients?

Fitness level

When we think of CF, we automatically think of lung & pancreatic problems. Which other body tissues are significantly affected by the disorder?
  (Name 3 tissues)

Liver (!)
Reproductive tract
Sweat glands

How is CF inherited?

Autosomal recessive

Which gene mutation is most important as a cause of CF?

Delta F508 –
A three base-pair deletion that eliminates a phenylalanine

Where is the cystic fibrosis gene located in the genome?

Chromosome 7 –
Long arm (same as "q")

The gene involved in CF is officially known as _____?

CFTR

(Cystic Fibrosis Transmembrane Receptor – at least this makes sense!)

Nasal polyps in a child <12 years old should make you consider what diagnosis?	CF – ¼ of all CF patients will have it!
CF patients very reliably have what ENT problem?	Pansinusitis
Lung structure & function are normal at birth for CF patients. Over time, what general category of pulmonary problem develops for them?	<u>Obstructive</u> pulmonary disease
What pattern of pulmonary function test (PFT) abnormalities is expected for CF patients? (Name 2 items)	• Decreased FEV1 & peak expiratory flow • Increased residual volume
Early in the course of CF, what infectious organisms most often bother the respiratory tract?	*Staph aureus* & Klebsiella (Pseudomonas/Burkholderia infection comes later)
What proportion of CF babies have pancreatic insufficiency *at birth*?	½
Only about 15 % of kids with CF have meconium ileus. What percentage will develop "meconium ileus equivalent" in childhood?	25 % (Same as "distal intestinal obstruction syndrome")
What is abnormal about the sweat produced by CF patients?	Very high sodium (& chloride) concentration
Other than providing a convenient way to test for CF, does the abnormality in sweat production have any clinical significance?	In infants, it can sometimes produce hyponatremia
What unusual joint finding suggests that your patient has CF?	Hypertrophic pulmonary osteoarthropathy Mnemonic: Thick secretions, Thick joints!

What joint & bone changes sometimes occur in CF, known as hypertrophic pulmonary osteo-arthropathy?

Periosteal thickening of long bones & their joints

In addition to meconium ileus & distal intestinal obstruction syndrome, what other GI problems can indicate a CF diagnosis?

Rectal prolapse
  Or
Intussusception in kids >1 year old

What impact does CF have on pubertal development?

Often delayed for both males & females

(due to nutrition/chronic illness issues)

What impact does CF have on male fertility?

The vas deferens is atretic –
in vitro fertilization is possible, but there are *no sperm in ejaculate*

What impact does CF have on female fertility?

Decreased fertility due to mucous abnormalities

How many mutations that produce CF have been identified so far?

>1,000!!!

(Less than 100 mutations produce 95 % of clinical disease, though)

When can a sweat test for CF be considered reliable?

If it is done by a CF center

Diagnosing CF requires that at least two criteria are met. There are two groups of criteria. What are they?
  (Name 3 items for each group)

(1st item – standard tests)
(2nd item – genetic factors)
(3rd item – clinical/unusual tests)

Group 1
1. + Newborn screen
2. CF in a sibling
3. Typical CF problems

Group 2
1. + Sweat test
2. + For two known CF mutations
3. + Nasal potential difference test

How is the newborn screening for CF done?

Blood test for IRT
(immunoreactive trypsinogen)

If a newborn screen for CF is positive, what does that mean?

Not much –
>90 % are false positives, so more tests are needed

If you suspect CF, and genetic testing reveals one CF mutation, how should you interpret that?

You can't –
4 % of the population carries CF genes (meaning has a single gene without disease)

Children with CF have the best chance for long-term survival when their care is provided by _____?

A CF center

What infectious diseases should prompt you to consider sweat testing, even though most of these kids will *not* turn out to have CF?
    (Name 2 diseases)

- **Pseudomonas or Burkholderia infection (other than otitis externa)**
- **Staph aureus pneumonia**

(Klebsiella is also concerning)

What ENT/respiratory issues should prompt you to consider sweat testing?
    (Name 4 issues)

- **Chronic cough or recurrent wheezing**
- **Pansinusitis**
- **Nasal polyps (<12 years old)**
- **Digital clubbing**

In addition to meconium ileus & rectal prolapse, what other GI issues should make you question whether CF might be the correct diagnosis?
    (Name 4 issues)

1. **Steatorrhea**
2. **Chronic diarrhea**
3. **Prolonged neonatal jaundice**
4. **Intussusception in kids older than 1 year**

Which types of exercise are most beneficial in CF?

Swimming & jogging

What are the mainstays of pulmonary treatment for CF?
    (Name 2 main modalities)

Antibiotics (various regimens)
    &
Chest PT/postural drainage
(one to four times daily)

If a CF patient has a pulmonary exacerbation, infection is usually involved. For moderate to severe exacerbations, what sort of treatment is usually required?

2–3 weeks IV antibiotics

If your CF patient is diagnosed with pseudomonal disease, which popular antibiotics must you *avoid* using?

Ceftriaxone –
Doesn't treat it!

A CF patient develops chest pain. She is afebrile, and has had the same problem before. What is the problem?

Pneumothorax

(10 % of CF patients develop this, and it often recurs)

How should hemoptysis be dealt with, in a CF patient?
  (Name 2 ways)

1. **Consider vitamin K if bleeding is brisk**

2. **Most CF bleeding is the result of infection – treat with antibiotics & withhold airway clearance during the acute phase**

What cardiac complication often develops late in the course of CF?

Pulmonary hypertension/
Cor pulmonale

If a CF patient develops clinical (right-sided) heart failure, what does this tell you about prognosis?

Survival <8 months is likely

(standard treatment is used – salt restriction, O_2, diuretics)

Is digitalis helpful, when treating the cardiac complications of CF?

No –
Not unless left-sided dysfunction is present

(not usually the case)

What medications are necessary to support gut absorptive function for CF patients? Why is absorption important to the pulmonary system?

• Pancreatic enzymes & H_2 blockers

• Normal height-to-weight ratios correlate with better pulmonary function

What other nutritional support is necessary for CF patients, if they are to maintain their height/weight ratio?
  (Name 2 items)

Extra vitamins A & E
High-fat diet

(Some kids also need nighttime enteral feeding)

CF patients are famous for having difficulties passing stool around the time of birth. What sort of difficulties do they tend to have with passing stool as they get older?

Diarrhea –
Usually foul-smelling & bulky

If CF patients often have diarrhea, why are they sometimes given Miralax® or other anti-constipation agents?

Constipation is even more common!

Which genotype is worst for α-1-antitrypsin deficiency?

Pi^{ZZ}

Although α-1-antitrypsin doesn't usually result in much pulmonary trouble in childhood, what body system is significantly affected, even in the young?

Liver –
Cirrhosis & hepatomas

When α-1-antitrypsin pulmonary problems present, what sort of problems do they have?

Emphysema (without smoking) in a young person –
Often with *bullous disease at the bases*

Patients who are heterozygous for α-1-antitrypsin will have what sort of pulmonary problems in their future?

None –
If they don't smoke

(If they smoke, they develop early disease!!!)

What sort of transplant will *prevent* α-1-antitrypsin pulmonary disease?

Liver transplant

How are α-1-antitrypsin patients treated for pulmonary problems?

Monthly infusions of the missing molecule *only when* pulmonary symptoms develop

(Note: There is no evidence that this helps)

What is alveolar proteinosis?

Overproduction of surfactant by confused alveolar macrophages!

How can alveolar proteinosis be treated?

Lavage the extra surfactant out
      &
Give GM-CSF
(sometimes gets the alveolar macrophages back on track)

Why does scleroderma cause pulmonary hypertension out of proportion to the pulmonary disease it causes (which is interstitial fibrosis)?

It causes proliferation of the intimal layer of the pulmonary artery → pulmonary hypertension

What are the main pulmonary effects of systemic lupus erythematosus?
(Name 3 effects)

Effusion
Pleuritis (painful)
Hemoptysis

What is the buzzword "noncaseating granuloma" associated with?

Sarcoid

What chest x-ray findings are expected in sarcoidosis?

Bilateral hilar lymphadenopathy

(sometimes mediastinal, also)

What sort of PFT findings are expected with sarcoidosis?

Restrictive

(& sometimes obstructive)

Which metabolic derangement is common with sarcoidosis?

Hypercalcemia
(& hypercalciuria)

How is sarcoidosis definitively diagnosed?

Biopsy showing noncaseating granuloma

What dermatological finding is a good sign in sarcoidosis?

Erythema nodosum

(purplish nodules, sometimes tender, on the shins)

Sarcoidosis clearly involves some derangement of the immune system. What are the typical abnormalities?
(Name 2 abnormalities)

1. **Hypergamma-globulinemia**
2. **>4:1 ratio of helper:suppressor T cells in fluid from BAL (bronchoalveolar lavage)**

What is the typical course for sarcoidosis in children?

75 % spontaneously recover

If sarcoidosis treatment is required, what is typically used?

Steroids
(improves symptoms, but doesn't induce remission)

Hypersensitivity pneumonitis also causes granulomas. What is the expected immune cell profile from BAL in this disorder?

<1:1 for helper:suppressor ratio

(*Suppressors are the bigger group, in other words*)

What is the most basic way to check that the pulse oximeter is functioning properly?

Check whether it is correlating correctly with the pulse

Chapter 4
Selected Cardiopulmonary Topics

Miliary Tuberculosis

Miliary tuberculosis occurs when massive bacteremia from a tuberculosis infection results in infection of multiple internal organs (at least two). The organs most often affected are the lungs, spleen, liver, and bone marrow. (Meningitis and peritonitis are also possibilities.)

Miliary tuberculosis usually develops 2–6 months after the initial infection, for those patients who are destined to develop it. *Most patients who develop miliary TB, though, do not have a known history of the disease.*

This disorder most commonly occurs in TB-infected infants and young children, although it is seen occasionally in adults. Children younger than 5 are more likely to develop life-threatening or meningeal involvement.

The onset is usually slow, although it can be sudden. There are two phases to the illness. Initially, the patient experiences fatigue and malaise and then later develops high fever, cough (may or may not be productive), lymphadenopathy, and hepato-splenomegaly. Over a period of several weeks, the lungs usually fill with foci of tubercular infection, called "tubers." This can result in respiratory distress and pneumothoraces.

The CXR will be normal in the early phases of miliary tuberculosis. Elderly patients often die of the disease before the chest X-ray shows any related abnormalities.

The most important factor in diagnosing miliary TB in children is a history of exposure to a tuberculosis-infected adult. Thirty percent of children with miliary tuberculosis will not test positive for TB. Alternatively, if an affected area, such as a lymph node, can be identified it can be biopsied for a definitive diagnosis.

Children respond well to treatment for miliary TB. Full recovery may take months, but they feel better within 2 weeks. The prognosis is less good for adults with miliary disease, but good outcomes are also possible if diagnosis and administration of the appropriate treatment are rapid.

C.M. Houser, *Pediatric Cardiology and Pulmonology: A Practically Painless Review*,
DOI 10.1007/978-1-4614-9481-2_4, © Springer Science+Business Media New York 2014

There is evidence to suggest that BCG vaccination protects children against developing miliary TB (and TB meningitis). This is the main reason to continue BCG vaccination for children in developing countries.

Sarcoid

Etiology

The cause of sarcoid is not at all clear. It is believed to be an undesirable immune response to some sort of environmental factor. In general, sarcoid is more common in colder areas than in warmer areas. Occasionally, clusters of sarcoid occur, indicating the importance of an environmental, or a local infectious, agent.

Interestingly, sarcoid sometimes forms in transplanted lungs, if the recipient previously had sarcoid. Even more disturbing, recipients of organs transplanted from sarcoid patients sometimes develop sarcoid!

In the United States, sarcoid is more common among African Americans. It is uncommon in children but can develop in adolescents.

Sarcoid: What Is It?

Non-caseating granulomas form in a variety of tissues – most commonly the lungs and hilar (near the lung hilum) lymph nodes. The clinical course of the disease is unpredictable – some people have very severe medical problems from sarcoid, while many sarcoid patients are actually asymptomatic.

Sarcoid patients who also develop erythema nodosum (raised, violaceous, tender plaques, usually on the anterior tibial area) usually have a good course with a full spontaneous recovery. *Bilateral hilar lymphadenopathy with erythema nodosum is termed **Lofgren's syndrome**.*

Sarcoid can affect almost any organ system. Its most serious effects result from damage to the lungs (pulmonary fibrosis, and honeycombing or cavity formation) and the heart (conduction/rhythm problems and heart failure). Sarcoid may also affect the skin, joints, eyes, and CNS. Hypercalcemia can also be seen with sarcoid.

Common presenting symptoms of sarcoid are dry cough, dyspnea on exertion, and intermittent chest pain, although the way it presents is highly variable. Children less than 8 years old tend to present with constitutional symptoms such as fever, fatigue, and weight loss. A subset of children presenting before their fourth birthday typically present with rash, arthritis, and uveitis.

Diagnosis

Although sarcoid can be diagnosed by biopsy, it is usually clinically diagnosed based on symptoms and the characteristic hilar lymphadenopathy appreciated on chest X-ray. Pulmonary function tests will show a restrictive pattern with reduction in DLCO (diffusion). Sarcoid is a diagnosis of exclusion; infectious granulomatous diseases caused by mycobacteria and fungus must be ruled out.

Treatment

There is no known treatment for sarcoid. To control symptoms, NSAIDs and steroids are most commonly used. Steroids have not been demonstrated to change the ultimate course of the disease – they just minimize the symptoms. In some cases, methotrexate has also been used to decrease symptoms and to minimize the amount of time the patient takes steroids. The ultimate prognosis for children who develop sarcoid is not well understood. Those who develop sarcoid before 4 years old appear to have a more complicated course.

Wegener's Granulomatosis (Granulomatosis with Polyangiitis) vs. Goodpasture's Disease

Wegener's Granulomatosis

Wegener's granulomatosis is a focal vasculitis. This means that it damages vessels in small, defined, areas – usually near the granulomas that it also produces. It mainly affects small vessels. The underlying cause of Wegener's is unknown, but patients usually test positive for antineutrophil cytoplasmic antibody (ANCA) and respond to immunosuppressive treatment, so autoimmune mechanisms are likely involved.

In the kidney, Wegener's causes a necrotizing glomerulonephritis that can present acutely, but sometimes presents more slowly. It is usually not present in children when they first present with the disorder. The *main effects* of Wegener's are in the lung and upper respiratory tract. Pulmonary involvement is always present in Wegener's. It causes a focal necrotizing vasculitis in the lung and upper airway, including the nose.

Patient presentation: Patients with Wegener's often present with nosebleeds, holes in the nasal septum (due to compromised blood flow from the vasculitic damage), and hemoptysis. They *are not* usually short of breath, because most of the lung parenchyma is unaffected but chronic cough and some dyspnea are common symptoms. Damage to the nasal septum can lead to "saddle nose" deformity.

Chest CT is important to confirm the diagnosis. Many patients eventually develop multi-organ involvement. They are also at increased risk for infection and sometimes develop resistant otitis media or sinusitis.

Treatment: Ninety percent of Wegener's patients respond well to immunosuppressive therapy. Typically, glucocorticoids and cyclophosphamide are used to induce initial remission, followed by methotrexate and azathioprine for maintenance therapy. Rituximab (monoclonal antibodies against B cells) is used as rescue therapy for those that don't respond to the usual initial treatment and for relapses.

It is fortunate that most Wegener's patients respond so well – without treatment, 80 % will die within a year of diagnosis.

Goodpasture's Disease

Goodpasture's is clearly an autoimmune disease. It results from the body producing antibodies against the basement membrane of the glomerulus. Unfortunately, these antibodies cross-react with the basement membrane of the alveoli, producing problems in both the kidney and the lung.

Patient presentation: Goodpasture's causes diffuse damage to the tissues in the kidney and the lungs. Goodpasture's causes *necrotizing, hemorrhagic, interstitial pneumonitis* and *acute glomerulonephritis*. Goodpasture's patients become significantly ill very quickly, after onset of the illness. *They have prominent dyspnea as part of their presentation.* Respiratory symptoms usually develop before the renal problems.

The "buzzword" for the histological appearance of Goodpasture's is:

"Continuous linear staining for IgG" along the basement membrane when immunofluorescent techniques are used

The patient's serum will also have antibody titers for anti-glomerular basement membrane (GBM) antibodies.

Treatment for Goodpasture's consists of steroids, cyclophosphamide, and sometimes plasmapheresis. Plasmapheresis usually produces great results initially, but most patients still go on to chronic renal failure.

Comparison

Wegener's

Nasal symptoms occur (epistaxis, septal damage)
Focal pathology – not diffuse
Vasculitic problem
Not usually short of breath

Cause unknown
Often ANCA +
Responds well to treatment
Prognosis good with treatment

Goodpasture's

Diffuse pathology (lungs and kidney)
Autoimmune problem
Antibody complex problem – visible on basement membranes
Short of breath at presentation
Response to treatment fair
Prognosis fair/chronic renal failure highly likely

Index

A

A-a gradient, 24, 25
ABG. *See* Arterial blood gas (ABG)
Acidosis, 23, 32–34, 47
Acute eosinophilic pneumonia, 48
Adenovirus pneumonia, 55
Albuterol, 40, 43
Alkalosis, 23, 32–34
Allergic bronchopulmonary aspergillosis, 48, 49, 69
Almitrine, 23
ALTE. *See* Apparent life-threatening event (ALTE)
Alveolar gas equation, 24–25
Alveolar hypoventilation, 25, 61
Alveolar proteinosis, 89
Alveoli, 23–25, 83, 94
Amoxicillin, 10
ANCA. *See* Antineutrophil cytoplasmic antibody (ANCA)
Anesthetics, 23
Antineutrophil cytoplasmic antibody (ANCA), 52, 53, 93, 95
Aorta, 1, 3, 4, 10, 18
Aortic coarctation, 3, 4
Aortic dissection, 6
Aortic valve, 1, 10, 18
Aortic valve stenosis, 1, 2, 10
Apnea, 30, 42, 43, 50, 57
Apparent life-threatening event (ALTE), 80, 81
ARDS, 38, 39, 83
Arrhythmia, 6, 7, 9, 17
Arterial blood gas (ABG), 8, 16, 24, 31–33, 39, 40, 42
Artificial valves, 12

Asphyxiating thoracic dystrophy, 62
Asthma, 27–31, 33–38, 41, 48, 49, 57, 58, 61, 71, 72, 75–77, 82
Asthma Predictive Index, 29
Asymptomatic hypertension, 4
Atelectasis, 43, 45, 82
Athletic heart, 3, 8
Atresia, 83
Atrial fibrillation, 7
Atrial flutter, 7, 9
Auscultatory exam, 12, 67
Autoimmune mechanisms, 93
AV block, 10
AV canal defect, 10

B

Bacterial endocarditis, 10, 11
BCG vaccination, 92
Beta-agonist, 22, 28, 37, 72
Bicarb, 32–34, 39
Bicuspid valves, 1
Bilateral hilar lymphadenopathy, 89, 92
Biopsy, 48, 53, 55, 64, 90, 91, 93
Blastomycosis, 69
Blood culture, 11, 66
Blunting, 23
BOOP. *See* Bronchiolitis obliterans organizing pneumonia (BOOP)
Bounding, 1, 13
BPD. *See* Bronchopulmonary dysplasia (BPD)
Bronchiectasis, 48, 49, 56, 57, 82
Bronchiolitis, 34, 41–44, 81
Bronchiolitis obliterans, 55, 56
Bronchiolitis obliterans organizing pneumonia (BOOP), 55, 56